SWEET DECEPTION

WHY SPLENDA®, NUTRASWEET®, AND THE FDA MAY BE HAZARDOUS TO YOUR HEALTH

DR. JOSEPH MERCOLA
WITH
DR. KENDRA DEGEN PEARSALL

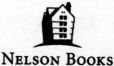

NELSON BOOKS
A Division of Thomas Nelson Publishers
Since 1798

www.thomasnelson.com

Copyright © 2006 by Dr. Joseph Mercola

Published in Nashville, Tennessee, by Thomas Nelson, Inc.

Nelson Books titles may be purchased in bulk for educational, business, fund-raising, or sales promotional use. For information, please e-mail SpecialMarkets@ThomasNelson.com.

Library of Congress Control Number: 2006932886

ISBN: 978-0-7852-9693-5

Printed in the United States of America

06 07 08 09 10 QW 5 4 3 2 1

KENDRA PEARSALL:

To Joe Mercola,
You have dedicated your entire life to your mission of waking people up to the corruption in our medical, food, and drug industries and to teaching people how to be naturally healthy. You have provided me with the inspiration and opportunities to work for this important mission. Since I met you in 2003, my life has been transformed in so many incredible ways, and I am forever grateful to you for taking me under your wing and showing me the positive changes one person can make for the good of the world.

To my mom, K'ana Degen,
You have always been my greatest source of unwavering love and support. Thank you for teaching me that being fearful and playing small does not serve the world and that my life is not just about me but about the difference I can make in the lives of others.

To an anonymous family member,
I've watched you eat very large quantities of artificial sweeteners every day for the past thirteen years. You went from being in perfect health to developing a long list of health problems including a neurological disease and depression. It is your suffering that inspired me to cowrite *Sweet Deception*. If this book is able to save just one person from ruining his or her health from artificial sweeteners, it will be worth it.

CONTENTS

FOREWORD

BEWARE OF STRANGERS
WITH SWEETS!

As parents, we warn our children, "Beware of strangers offering you candy and sweets!" We tell our sons and daughters, "Run the other way!" if any stranger even starts to insist they accept the sweets. Most of our children heed this lesson. A few give in to temptation and may pay a very heavy price for the mistake.

As adults, we don't even think that most of the strangers—in this case, giant corporations—who offer us "sweets" may also not have our best interests in mind. While the harm these corporate "strangers" will do to us if we give in to their sweet temptation usually isn't as immediate as what befalls unwary children, over time it can still be serious, and isn't always reversible.

In this long-needed book, very aptly titled *Sweet Deception,* Drs. Mercola and Pearsall and their team document the enormous range of health problems—some temporary, some permanent—caused by both patented chemical sweeteners and highly refined sugar.

Just one of these patented chemicals has been found to cause seizures and loss of vision, headaches, vomiting, diarrhea, memory loss, visual impairment, weight gain, increased cancer risk, and even death—and literally dozens of symptoms more. If we include other patented chemical sweeteners and highly refined sugars, the list of health impairments linked to them is staggering.

So why are these toxic chemicals allowed in our nation's food? And why aren't "health authorities" and government agencies warning us about them via the media? After all, in just the first few months of 2006, we were warned—based on poorly done or even bogus studies—that calcium and vitamin D don't help our bones, that we're wasting our money on glucosamine for arthritis, that saw palmetto doesn't really help all those men whose prostate symptoms it obviously improved; the year before, we were warned that vitamin E might kill us.

So why haven't we been treated to similar publicity about the very real dangers of patented chemical sweeteners as well as the highly refined natural ones?

As experienced adults, we're instantly on guard when we hear the phrase: "We're from the government, we're here to help." But we're not yet fully "grown up" about the ways of government and its innumerable agencies. We must learn that government is just as likely to be deceiving us when it's silent on a topic as when they're talking about it. Who hasn't read that pregnant women shouldn't eat tuna because mercury will hurt the baby, while nothing at all is said about pregnant women getting mercury-containing dental amalgams, which release much more mercury into the baby than any tuna ever could? A dental amalgam releases 10 mcg per filling per day, and a can of tuna contains 20 mcg of mercury.[1,2]

As stated by Food and Drug Administration insiders themselves, documented here by Drs. Mercola and Pearsall, the giant food processing industries and patent medicine companies are FDA's "clients" to be protected, *not you and me!* The very agency that's charged by Congress with "protecting" your health, the FDA, does not believe their "client" is the American people![3]

But this is nothing new. In 1970, former FDA commissioner Herbert Ley was quoted in print: "People think the FDA is protecting them—it isn't. What the FDA is doing and what people think it's doing are as different as night and day."[4]

In testimony before Congress, FDA commissioner Charles Edwards said, "[It is] not our [FDA] policy to jeopardize the financial interests of the pharmaceutical companies."[5] Even worse, the FDA not only works to protect "Big Pharma" and "agri-business," it actively fights good health practices, and has done so for generations.

In 1949, FDA commissioner George Larrick said, "The activities of . .

. so called health food lecturers have increasingly engaged our attention . . . [we are] fighting the good fight against dried vegetables, mineral mixtures, vitamins, and similar products."[6]

According to former U.S. senator Edward V. Long, "If the FDA would spend a little less time and effort on small manufacturers of vitamins . . . and a little more on manufacturers of . . . dangerous drugs . . . the public would be better served."[7] In fact, hundreds of books, including this one, document beyond any doubt that government is not to be believed when it says it's "protecting your health."

The FDA is protecting its "clients" (mostly giant corporations), and giant corporations are busy protecting their profits . . . and those profits are greatest if they're selling you a patented chemical. (Profits are also very good on unpatentable but highly refined sugars.) Whether or not those chemicals or highly refined sugars are good for your health is a remotely second-place concern to the "strangers" in those giant corporations. Their concern is limited to protecting their profits by not killing you or giving you immediately recognizable symptoms, so you'll keep on buying the product!

If you haven't learned already that only you truly care about your health and the health of your family, it's time to grow up! It's up to you to investigate and make your own decisions about what's best for your health. Even your trusted family doctor (who, after you, probably cares more about your health than anyone) has all too often bought the food industry/FDA "line" about the supposed safety of chemical sweeteners and highly refined sugars. Quick test: has he or she warned you not to use them?

Please read this book! Then, if you value your health, follow every parent's advice to his or her children, but this time with another dimension of understanding: "Beware of strangers offering sweets!"

—JONATHAN V. WRIGHT, MD
Medical Director, Tahoma Clinic, Renton, Washington
Author of *Natural Hormone Replacement for Women Over 45*
(with Lane Lenard, PhD), and
*Natural Healing, Optimal Wellness: The Patient's Guide to
Health and Healing* (with Alan R. Gaby, MD)

INTRODUCTION
SWEET TALK

WHY YOU SHOULD READ THIS BOOK

All truth passes through three stages
- *First it is ridiculed*
- *Then it is violently opposed*
- *Finally, it is accepted as self-evident.*
                    —*Arthur Schopenhouer (1788–1860)*
                              German philosopher

You see the little packets of artificial sweeteners laid out for you whenever you go to a restaurant. There they are in pink, blue, and yellow—the colors of baby clothes. Friendly colors. You know they've been approved by the Food and Drug Administration (FDA) and that some of them have been around for decades. They're in all your diet sodas and snacks. But still, you're not entirely sure about them. There's a nagging question at the back of your mind when you see them. *Are these really safe?*

You are right to ask that question. The answer is no.

The Current Epidemic

Seventy million Americans suffer from some form of cardiovascular disease. Twenty million have diabetes, and forty-five million are prediabetic. An overwhelming 65 percent of U.S. adults are overweight, and 30 percent are obese. We are seeing strokes, cancers, Alzheimer's, and autism in record numbers, and those numbers are climbing.

It wasn't always like this.

Artificial sweeteners are not the only cause of these problems, of course. But they are one of them—and this book will clearly tell you exactly how and why. And they are worth singling out, because they are, in a way, emblematic of everything that's gone wrong with the diet of industrialized nations, everything that is causing this great plague of multiple diseases. Artificial sweeteners are just about the worst of all possible worlds, as far as dietary choices go: they are completely unnatural, insufficiently tested for safety, unnecessary in the diet, and have a long history of causing health problems. They are powerful examples of a diet gone mad.

The FDA Will Not Protect You

Many believe that artificial sweeteners cannot possibly be as bad as all that; after all, they have been declared safe by the FDA, the government organization that is there to protect us from just such a threat. But the FDA, I'm sorry to say, has been unable to protect the public for quite some time.

Vioxx was a drug that hit the marketplace with great fanfare in 1999. It was FDA-approved for safety and heavily promoted to physicians and patients by Merck, the company that made it. Five years later, it was withdrawn after having been implicated in the deaths of over sixty thousand people. The FDA had failed the public.

Yet a few months after the recall, the FDA voted to allow Vioxx to go back on the market *again*. The FDA has failed a *second* time, with a drug it knows is dangerous. What's going on?

The truth of the matter is, structural and organizational changes to the FDA over the last few decades, prompted by big business and passed by a heavily lobbied Congress, have left it a pawn of the very industries it was designed to regulate. The specifics of the changes and their implications will be covered in detail within this book, but for now it's enough to know: the FDA is no longer protecting you. All that it protects now are the profits of its multinational corporation "clients."

Questions That Need Answers

The questions regarding the safety of artificial sweeteners come in many forms. Many people are trying to piece together what's really going on from a collection of half-heard rumors, industry denials, biased commercials, and unreliable sources. Not knowing all of the facts, you wonder: *Didn't they find out NutraSweet® caused migraine headaches or something like that? Whatever happened to those cancer warnings that used to come with saccharin? Has Splenda® really been tested enough?* You wonder how concerned you should be about your health, or even if you should be concerned at all.

Many people who want to know the real answers contact me through my natural health Web site, Mercola.com. I've received thousands of inquiries about the safety of artificial sweeteners, asking such things as:

- Is Splenda really as safe as they claim it is?

- Is Splenda really natural sugar?

- What are the long-term risks of consuming artificial sweeteners?

- Do artificial sweeteners cause cancer?

- Do they affect your nervous system or brain?

- How does Splenda affect diabetics, your risk of diabetes, or your insulin levels?

- Are artificial sweeteners safe for children and pregnant women?

- Can they cause allergic reactions?

- Do they really help you lose weight?

- What is the inside scoop on why the FDA approves dangerous drugs and food additives?

- What are the safe alternatives to artificial sweeteners? Is stevia safe?

- What's the difference between Splenda and aspartame?

- Which is worse for you, artificial sweeteners or sugar?

This book addresses these and other questions. You will find that the answers are almost universally disturbing: artificial sweeteners, are among the worst "foods" you can put in your body. They can cause serious illnesses, weaken your immune system, and make you susceptible to yet more diseases . . . and, as it turns out, they don't even really help you lose weight.

To fully answer all of the questions, we'll look at the motives and practices of the multinational corporations that make and sell artificial sweeteners. We'll examine the disastrous structural changes at the FDA we previously mentioned. We'll investigate the possibility of biases in scientific studies, the reliability of assurances that artificial sweeteners are safe, and the trustworthiness of the sources of such information. We'll also go over some basic biochemistry to help you understand the chemical structures of various artificial sweeteners, as well as sugar itself.

Along the way, you'll hear the real stories of people who have had their health damaged by artificial sweeteners. You'll also find out about behind-the-scenes political deals, accidental discoveries, dangerous environmental pollution, shoddy science, and deceptive advertising.

I think, after reading all of the information, you'll find yourself agreeing with me that artificial sweeteners are to be avoided at all costs.

Cutting Through the Deception

But this book doesn't end with that. It goes further, to examine what a healthy diet actually consists of and the real place of sweeteners in your diet. Some of that information may surprise you. But if you choose to accept it, you may find yourself not only wanting to avoid sweeteners because of their dangers but having no need or desire for their taste as well.

My ultimate goal is that you more fully appreciate the benefits of a healthy, natural diet—the kind your body was designed for and that your ancestors enjoyed. Your body did not evolve by eating synthetic chemicals, processed sugars, irradiated and genetically altered foods, pesticide-doused plants, hormone-laden meats, and all the other chemical "wonders" that modern technology has provided. You are now regularly tempted with a cheap, abundant supply of convenient and tasty processed foods that are slowly killing you. Your body works best when you provide it with foods as they were originally found in nature, as your distant ancestors ate them for many thousands of years—certainly long before a series of accidental chemical spills gifted us with the first artificial sweeteners.

It is my sincere expectation that reading this book will help you understand how you have been manipulated by industries whose primary focus is to increase their profits, and that have careless disregard for the health of you and your family.

You don't have to stand for this behavior anymore.

CHAPTER ONE:
SWEET TOOTH

SUGAR—WHAT IT IS, WHY YOU CRAVE IT, AND HOW IT'S KILLING YOU

Our ancestors were primarily hunter-gatherers. They did not farm; they simply ate the pure, natural foods that they could find in their environment such as meats, fish, fruits, vegetables, nuts, and seeds. And they had the lowest body fat to total body weight ratio of any people in the history of the world.

Your ancient ancestors had excellent muscle tone and physical fitness. If they survived the hazards of infectious disease, trauma, and childbirth, they had a life span comparable to what we have today. When we examine their remains, we see little evidence that they suffered from our contemporary chronic degenerative diseases, such as obesity, diabetes, heart disease, cancer, tooth decay, arthritis, and osteoporosis.[1]

Our modern mythology portrays life in that era as a never-ending, physically punishing struggle to survive. But in fact, anthropological studies show that hunter-gatherers did not burn many more calories in a day than they would have playing a leisurely round of golf.[2] At the same time, they ate far more food than the typical American living today. So they ate *more*, exercised *less*, and were healthier and more physically fit. What was going on?

There are still a few hunter-gatherer cultures that exist to the present day. Dr. Weston Price, a prominent researcher, studied these societies of the early twentieth century, and spent a lifetime documenting his findings in his landmark book, *Nutrition and Physical Degeneration*, initially published in 1939 and now in its seventeenth edition.[3] He found a nearly complete absence of chronic degenerative disease among the hunter-gatherers. He also observed that as these cultures switched from their hunter-gatherer diet to a more industrialized diet of processed foods, they fell prey to the same high rates of degenerative diseases as the industrialized cultures.

It seems they, like the rest of the modern world, had become addicted to sugar.

A Cure Worse than the Disease

Modern man consumes sugar in vast quantities. We crave the taste, while at the same time we are at least somewhat aware that our dietary habits are killing us. If nothing else, we have at least heard the well-publicized risks associated with high sugar consumption and obesity. This is just the tip of the iceberg.

Artificial sweeteners—products like saccharin, aspartame (NutraSweet), and sucralose (Splenda)—may seem at first glance to be an ideal solution to the problem. Their sweet taste satisfies our desire for sugar, while their lack of calories makes them sound like healthier alternatives. It seems like a win-win situation, but it isn't.

In fact artificial sweeteners could be more dangerous than sugar itself. Instead of being a cure for our addiction, they are simply another drug—an even worse one.

Sugar, Sugar

To fully understand artificial sweeteners, we need to start by looking at sugar itself. Without your desire for sugar, after all, there would be no need for anything to replace it. And an examination of the health risks of sugar will amply demonstrate why we are so desperate for something less dangerous to replace it—something that does not exist, although businesses are happy to claim it does, and sell us the dangerous chemicals discussed throughout this book.

The Origins of Sweeteners

The only concentrated sugar that early man would have had access to was honey. But observational research of modern-day hunter-gatherers shows that the average honey consumption was minor—maybe four pounds, or 3 percent of total calories, over the course of an entire year.[4,5] It was not until 500 A.D. that the Indians introduced mass sugar extraction by pressing out the juice out of sugarcane and boiling it into crystals. For many centuries, sugar production was labor intensive, and therefore expensive to produce. This effectively restricted the use of sugar to all but the very wealthy.

But the sugar industry experienced a revolutionary shift after Christopher Columbus arrived in the New World. When Columbus sailed to the Caribbean islands in 1492, he planted sugarcane, which thrived in the favorable climate. In modern America, we tend to think of cotton plantations as the driving economic force behind slavery. But in fact, historical documents make it quite clear that without sugar, the slave trade would have been relatively minor. African slavery was the main factor that radically changed the economics of the sugar industry and was able to reduce the cost of sugar from the $100 per kilo 1319 price to the equivalent of $6 per kilo by 1500. Finally, sugar was inexpensive enough for the average person to use. Between 1663 and 1775, English use of sugar increased twentyfold, and nearly all of it was produced in the Americas.

In the years that followed, the costs of sugar production continued to plummet, causing consumption to dramatically increase. Over the course of the nineteenth century, the English would up their sugar consumption once again, this time fivefold.[6]

A more complete history of sugar is available in appendix E.

The Advent of High-Fructose Modified Corn Syrup

In 1968, there was a revolutionary breakthrough in the sweetener industry when new technology made it economically feasible to manufacture mass quantities of high-fructose corn syrup (HFCS) and the similar hydrolyzed high-fructose inulin syrup. Being a liquid, HFCS is easier to dissolve in other liquids, and it is twenty times sweeter than cane sugar, meaning smaller (and therefore cheaper) amounts can be used.

HFCS is now nearly the exclusive caloric sweetener used in the soft-drink industry, and it is also used in juice, condiments, jams, and wine, but is not available for home use. Presently, HFCS dominates the sweetener industry, accounting for 55 percent of the market and $4.5 billion in annual sales. In 2003, Americans consumed sixty-one pounds of HFCS per person.[7]

So, What Is Sugar?

To understand what sugar is, we have to cover a few nutritional basics. All food can be classified into three basic types of macronutrients: carbohydrates, fats, and proteins. Each nutrient type provides an important function for your body:

Functions of Macronutrients

CARBOHYDRATES	PROTEINS	FATS
Energy source	Energy source	Energy source
	Build tissue and bone	Protect organs
	Transport molecules	Transport nutrients
	Blood pressure	Body temperature
	pH balance	Hormone synthesis

As you can see from this table, the only function of carbohydrates is to provide your body with energy. But since protein and fat can also provide energy, carbohydrates are not essential for your survival. (Sugar is a form of carbohydrates.) On the other hand, if your body does not receive enough protein or fat, you will perish.

Carbohydrates are classified into two types: simple and complex. Complex carbohydrates consist of polysaccharides (long chains of mono- or disaccharides), which include starch, cellulose, and/or fiber. Sugars are simple carbohydrates (monosaccharides and disaccharides by themselves). With the exception of honey, the carbohydrate foods found in nature are complex carbohydrates, or a combination of complex and simple carbohydrates. But when natural foods are processed, the complex carbs are frequently removed. For example, an apple ordinarily contains both, but when it is juiced and its fiber is removed, the juice contains only simple carbohydrates.

Because simple carbohydrates are rapidly absorbed into your bloodstream, they cause large spikes in blood sugar that can contribute to obesity, heart disease, cancer, and diabetes.

Monosaccharides

A monosaccharide is the simplest form of sugar, from which all complex carbohydrates are formed. The three monosaccharides of nutritional importance are glucose (dextrose), galactose, and fructose.

Glucose—This monosaccharide provides energy to all the tissues of your body. It is also known as "blood sugar."

Galactose—This monosaccharide is found in lactose or milk sugar and is important in the production of healthy intestinal flora in your gut.

Fructose—This monosaccharide is also called "fruit sugar" because it is found in fruit (as well as in honey). It is the sweetest of the natural sugars.

Disaccharides

Disaccharides are doubled monosaccharides. They require enzymes to be broken down into monosaccharides for digestion.

Sucrose (table sugar) is composed of fructose and glucose.

Maltose is composed of two glucose molecules.

Lactose is composed of glucose and galactose.[8]

(You'll notice that all three natural disaccharides contain glucose. This will become important when we get to our discussion of Splenda in chapter 4.)

Why You Love Sugar

With 115 million tons of sugar currently being produced each year, it seems safe to say that nearly the entire world has an insatiable appetite for it. Dr. Daniel Kirschenbaum, a weight loss expert, offers two reasons why we are born with such a powerful sweet tooth:

> When you are hungry, sugar provides the quickest antidote . . . When people or other animals are starving, they consistently show heightened preferences for very sweet foods. This, again, shows your body's orientation to satisfy extreme hunger and food deprivation quickly and effectively with sugar.

Sweet foods are safe foods. Can you think of any examples of wild fruits or berries or vegetables that are sweet and also dangerous to eat? Probably not. If you find something hanging from a tree and it tastes sweet, it is almost certainly safe to eat. On the other hand, sour or bitter fruits or vegetables are much more likely to be poisonous.[9]

Your body is programmed to eat large amounts of sugar or sweet foods whenever they are available. This made sense for our hunter-gatherer ancestors; if they found something that tasted sweet, their bodies wanted to encourage them to eat large quantities of it.

The innate desire for sweets has been observed in primitive societies like the Aborigines of Australia and the Bushmen of South Africa, who undergo great efforts to seek raw honey and consume high amounts whenever they can find it. However "high amounts" for them means about *4 pounds* per person per year—unlike the typical American who at the turn of this last century was eating an estimated *158 pounds* of sugar per year.[10]

The addiction is very real. Research studies indicate that sugar may be similar to morphine and heroin in its ability to increase opioids in your brain that produce pleasure. This increase in opioids is a major part of the physiology that fuels your addiction and the craving for sugar, which is why the sugar consumption rates are climbing each year.[11]

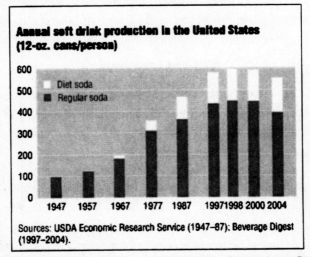

Reprinted, with permission, from "Liquid Candy," Center for Science in the Public Interest.[12]

**Amount of Caloric Sweeteners Consumed
per Person in the United states**

- 1880: 38 lb.
- 1970: 119 lb.
- 1990: 132 lb.
- 2005: 149 lb. = 1 cup/day

But your natural craving for sugar is not the only factor in this. Another cause is the marketing and advertising that goes into promoting sugar-laden foods. TV commercials promoting junk food loaded with sugar seem to permeate children's programming. Both Pepsi™ and Coca-Cola™ make large donations to public schools in order to establish exclusive marketing rights. Soft-drink manufacturers license their logos to baby bottles because the research shows that parents are much more likely to feed their infant with their brand of soda if the bottle has their logo on it.[13]

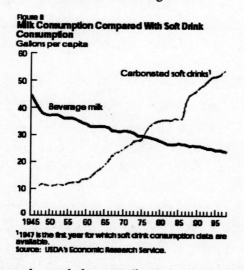

Figure 8
Milk Consumption Compared With Soft Drink Consumption
Gallons per capita

Carbonated soft drinks[1]

Beverage milk

[1]1947 is the first year for which soft drink consumption data are available.
Source: USDA's Economic Research Service.

Feeding newborns soda pop helps contribute to a very strong sugar dependency. These newborns typically mature into children who constantly plead with their parents for more sugar and soft drinks to satisfy their insatiable cravings. Since the late seventies, one-fifth of toddlers have been given eight ounces of soda every day, and almost half of all children between the ages of six and eleven have drunk an average of fifteen ounces per day. However, the heavyweight soda pop drinkers are teenagers, who gulp between twenty-three and thirty ounces per day.[14]

In the 1950s, the standard serving of Coca-Cola was a 6.5-ounce bottle and was used as an occasional treat. Soft drinks have now progressed to being the number one source of sugar in the American diet. In 2004, 15.3 billion gallons of soft drinks were sold in the United States—the equivalent of about one and a half 12-ounce cans of soda pop per day for every American citizen.[15] And over time, the size of the bottle has increased from 6.5 ounces to 12, then 20, and now 64-ounce Big Gulps® (with eight hundred calories and fifty-three teaspoons of sugar).[16]

The fact that there is so much *hidden* sugar in the food supply further contributes to our ever-increasing sugar intake. You probably are not aware that most processed food products contain sugar; even products you would not suspect to contain sugar are loaded with it. This includes items like meat, hamburgers, canned salmon, bouillon cubes, luncheon meats, nuts, alcohol, cereals, peanut butter, soups, sauces, dressings, medications, baked goods, frozen dinners . . . the list goes on and on. The food manufacturers use sugar as a cheap bulking agent and flavor enhancer.

Confessions of a Teenaged Sugar Junkie

I (Pearsall) remember clearly what the gastronomic culture was like when I attended high school from 1987 to 1991. During lunch it was considered "cool" to just get a quick snack at the snack line because most of the kids who went through the hot lunch line were poor and had sub-sized lunch tickets. Every day I would scan the lunchroom and look at the rows and rows of people eating their purchases from the snack line: chocolate chip cookies, sweetened yogurt, orange juice, soft pretzels, potato chips, and french fries with lots of catsup. I'm embarrassed to admit that I would buy this kind of food at times just because I was so desperate to fit in with everyone else.

Another "in" thing to do was to drive to 7-11 after school and buy a Big Gulp and some candy. In fact I have no memory of seeing anyone drink water in high school; soda pop, juice, and of course alcohol were the socially accepted beverages to drink. In speaking with teenagers in the twenty-first century, it appears things have only worsened on the nutritional scene. Given the yearly increases of sugar consumption and obesity among kids and adolescents, it seems there is no end in sight to this nutritional nightmare. In fact, experts now predict that for the first time in history, the current generation of children will not outlive their parents due to their poor diets.

Our unlimited access to sugar, combined with our inherent desire for sweet foods (and the constant barrage from the food industry to convince us to satisfy our cravings), has led many of us to consume as much sugar in one week as our ancestors did in an entire year. We eat sugar at every meal. We celebrate with sugar. We reward our kids with sugar. We sell sugar-laden foods to our kids in the school cafeterias. We begin our workday with sugary pastries in the staff lounges. We serve dessert after dinner. Unfortunately, there are serious consequences for this type of abuse.

Western nations are in the midst of the worst obesity epidemic to ever hit the planet. There are record numbers of cancers, heart attacks, strokes, and Alzheimer's disease. One of the primary culprits is our craving for sugar, combined with the convenience and affordability of many processed foods that contain it.

The Many Problems with Sugar

Using the search terms *sugar* and *harm* on Google gives more than six million links about the harmful effects of sugar. So you probably realize that sugar is bad for you—but you might be unable to list all the specific reasons why.

Sugar Increases Insulin and Contributes to Obesity and Diabetes

One of the most important points to understand about sugar is the effect it has on your physiology. If you were to take all of the sugar that is in the one gallon of blood circulating in your body, there would be only about one teaspoon's worth. So let's say, for example, you drink a glass of orange juice, which contains eight teaspoons of sugar and water. The sugar in the juice travels into your stomach, and then into your intestine, where it is rapidly absorbed into your bloodstream because there is no fiber to inhibit its absorption process. But if the eight teaspoons of sugar from the juice were absorbed into your bloodstream unmetabolized, you would rapidly go into a hyperglycemic coma and die.

However, your pancreas saves the day and quickly secretes large amounts of insulin to process the onslaught of sugar. While this prevents you from dying in the short run, if this process is repeated in a frequency that is consistent with the diet of most Americans, your insulin levels will be regularly elevated. This will kill you in the long run with the development of a chronic disease such as weight gain, heart disease, or cancer.

Insulin is a hormone that binds to receptors on your cells in order to activate glucose transporters that grab the sugar molecules and bring them inside your cells. Your cells have a limited capacity for sugar to enter, and any excess will be stored as fat. Not only is insulin a fat-building hormone, but when secreted in excess (as in the case of eating a high amount of carbohydrates) it also increases your cholesterol, increases blood pressure, and causes thickening of the lining of your arteries. This contributes to heart disease—in fact, the primary predictor of heart disease is high insulin levels.[17] Without a doubt the best way to prevent aging and degenerative disease is to keep your insulin levels in a low but healthy range. Every year, billions of dollars are spent in the antiaging industry when the most effective (and inexpensive) thing you can do to slow the aging process is keep your insulin levels normal by restricting

OBESITY-RELATED COMPLICATIONS

- Decreased life span
- Heart disease and stroke
- High blood pressure and cholesterol
- Diabetes
- Cancer
- Gallbladder disease and gallstones
- Osteoarthritis
- Gout
- Breathing problems, snoring, sleep apnea (when a person stops breathing for a short time during sleep), and asthma
- Depression

your intake of grains and sugars and engaging in sufficient cardiovascular exercise.

Overconsumption of sugar over time can cause your pancreas to "burn out" from having to secrete large amounts of insulin. Normally, your body has stored insulin that can be secreted immediately when you eat sugar. But with high sugar consumption, this stored insulin is rapidly used up, and it may be hours before your pancreas can make enough insulin to bring your blood sugars back down to normal. High blood sugar levels are dangerous, because the longer the glucose molecules are free floating in your blood, the higher the chance they will attach to cell proteins and damage them, resulting in what is known as advanced glycation end products (AGEs), which can cause your tissues and organs to degenerate.[18]

At the same time, sustained high insulin levels can lead to insulin resistance. If your cells are stuffed with fat and sugar, they cannot respond appropriately to insulin. This forces your pancreas to make many times the normal amount of insulin in an effort to stimulate your cells to respond. The result is a vicious cycle; the high insulin causes some of your sugar to be stored as fat, the increased body fat causes insulin resistance, and the insulin resistance prevents your glucose from entering your cells. So you still feel hungry and eat more, which causes your pancreas to work even harder to produce more insulin, which triggers the vicious cycle of even more weight gain, increased insulin resistance, and eventual pancreas cell burnout leading to severe diabetes.

Anyone who is overweight, is diabetic, has high cholesterol, or has ever had elevated fasting blood sugars is best served by having their fasting insulin levels tested, because *one in three Americans is insulin resistant.* You can learn about the blood tests for fasting blood sugar and insulin in chapter 8. Insulin resistance causes weight gain and can make weight loss very difficult. And resolving insulin resistance is one of the

COMPLICATIONS OF DIABETES

- Retinopathy, blindness
- Cardiovascular disease
- Stroke
- Neuropathy
- Impotence
- Kidney failure
- Overweightness, obesity
- Gastroparesis (poor food digestion)
- Premature death

most important steps in treating diabetes, so it is imperative to follow the guidelines in chapter 8 if you are insulin resistant.

The reason low-carb diets help you lose weight is because they keep your insulin levels low. When you keep your insulin levels low, you maximize your fat-burning enzymes and are able to burn your fat stores as an alternative energy source to carbohydrates.

Sugar Causes You to Lose Important Minerals

Studies have shown that sugar depletes the minerals in your body. For example, it disrupts your calcium-phosphorus ratio (optimally 10:4) by increasing your rate of calcium excretion. When you increase your calcium excretion, your body needs to compensate for this by removing the calcium from your bones to buffer this loss, and this can lead to osteoporosis. Unfortunately, simply taking calcium supplements can cause you more harm than good, as the rest of the minerals may not be in proper balance. Your body is constantly trying to maintain homeostasis, as disease can result from even slight deviations from optimal mineral and pH balance. These delicate mineral ratios are disturbed with as little as two teaspoons of sugar, and if sugar is ingested on a regular basis, your body may lose its ability to restore the balance on its own—which leads to disease.

Sugar Disturbs Your Hormones

Your endocrine system is composed of a number of interconnected glands that secrete hormones that serve as messengers for bodily functions. When you eat sugar, some of your glands are forced to work hard to compensate for the unhealthy effects that sugar has on your body. For example, your adrenal gland, sitting on top of your kidneys, is excessively stimulated when you eat sugar. This can weaken your adrenals. Your adrenals play a role in sodium and potassium regulation, blood pressure, glucose metabolism, and cortisol, adrenaline, and sex steroid secretion (DHEA, testosterone, and estrogen). It is very common for adrenal fatigue to cause serious health problems. You may want to look at the list below to see if you have any of the signs of weakened adrenal glands. If so, it is even more important that you seriously consider a program to radically reduce or eliminate your use of sugar.

Symptoms of Weakened Adrenals

Allergies	Arthritis
Asthma	Candida
Chronic fatigue syndrome	Degenerative disease of aging
Depression	Fatigue (most common symptom)
Headaches	Insomnia
Irritable bowel syndrome	Mental exhaustion
Susceptible to infections	Short emotional fuse (easily angry or weepy)

Sugar Can Lead to Food Allergies

To be digested and assimilated into your cells, food has to be broken down by enzymes. Enzymes function best when your body has the appropriate mineral balance. When you eat sugar, your mineral stores become depleted, and this compromises your enzyme function that allows undigested food particles to enter your bloodstream. When this happens, your immune system can confuse food particles as foreign invaders, signaling your body to launch an attack whenever you eat that food. This can cause acute reactions such as rashes, sleepiness, or joint pain.

But even worse, if you regularly eat this food, it may cause your body to adapt without these reactions. This may happen because your immune system becomes weakened from constantly having to mount a defense against the allergenic food. Your exhausted immune system predisposes you to many chronic degenerative diseases. Food allergies clearly affect the majority of people, but very few are ever able to associate their symptoms with what they are eating, because conventional medicine and the general public are largely unaware of food allergies.[19]

Sugar Paralyzes Your Immune System

Phagocytes are types of white blood cells that engulf foreign bacteria and viruses, and are an integral part of your immune system. They serve important roles in preventing and controlling infections from bacteria and viruses. Studies conducted at Loma Linda University showed that the number of organisms eaten by phagocytes decreased dramatically for up to six hours after eating sugar.[20] Do you really want to weaken your immune system for six hours? Even if you are unable to stop your sugar addiction, one of the key take-home messages here is that if you are just coming down with an infection, or already have one, one of the worst things you can do is eat sugar. It is nearly guaranteed to prolong your illness by seriously sabotaging your immune system.

Sugar Intake Leads to Chronic Diseases

In 1986, the Food and Drug Administration (FDA) issued a report on American sugar consumption and its harmful effects on health. One of the conclusions (based on published studies) was that diets containing 25 percent or more of their calories as sugar could result in one or more of the following:

- Diabetes
- Hypoglycemia
- Cardiovascular disease
- Behavioral problems
- Mineral deficiencies
- Gallstones

The implication is that Americans need to cut down on their sugar intake if they want to avoid disease. Unfortunately, the FDA gave Americans a false sense of security with their final conclusion—that Americans need not worry about their diets because nobody eats that much sugar.[21] This is patently false; the per capita consumption in 1999 was 158 pounds, which would have been anywhere from 20 to 40 percent of the caloric intake.

One of the ways that a high sugar intake can cause degenerative diseases is that high levels of sugar in your bloodstream attach to your proteins in a way that causes permanent harm to their molecular structure. These damaged proteins are the advanced glycation end products (AGEs) that were mentioned earlier, and they can cause cell destruction and chronic degenerative diseases such as Alzheimer's, cataracts, arthritis, and heart disease. You should also know that AGEs are not only caused by high sugar intake but also by browning foods (toasting bread, baking meat, broiled potatoes, baking cookies, etc.), because the browning occurs when the glucose attaches to the protein in your food.[22] Therefore, it is best to eat foods raw, steamed, or cooked in water to keep intake of AGEs to a minimum.

Sugar Increases Your Cancer Risk

In early 2005, cancer finally passed heart disease as the number one cause of death in the United States. Many scientists and medical specialists have proposed that sugar intake can lead to cancer by the following mechanism: The cells of your body naturally produce waste products called free radicals. Your body compensates with enzymes to neutralize the toxic effects of these free radicals. These protective enzymes require the proper mineral balance in order to be effective, and since sugar drains the minerals of your body, your enzymes are not nearly as effective as they could be. This leads to a buildup of free radicals, which then can cause a decrease in the availability of oxygen to your cells that can lead to cancerous cell mutations.[23] This correlates with research done by Dr. Otto Walberg in the 1920s that showed that cells became cancerous when 35 percent of the oxygen was removed from their environment.

If all the harmful effects of sugar that I've listed so far aren't convincing enough, appendix A has a list of seventy-six ways that sugar can destroy your health.

HFCS causes all of the negative effects of other sugars and more. When you eat fructose in its natural state, as in fruit, it is less likely to cause a problem. As long as you are not struggling with diabetes, obesity, or yeast problems, one to two pieces of fruit a day will likely improve your health. But high consumption of processed fructose such as HFCS can cause problems, since the digestion, absorption, and metabolism of fructose differ from those of glucose in disadvantageous ways.

> **HFCS CAN CAUSE THE FOLLOWING HEALTH PROBLEMS:**
> - Weight gain
> - Accelerated bone loss
> - Insulin resistance
> - Glucose intolerance
> - High cholesterol and triglycerides
> - High blood pressure (animal studies)
> - Liver damage (animal studies)
> - Increased risk for AGEs, mineral loss, and oxidative damage

First, when your liver processes fructose, it stimulates fat production, and therefore can cause weight gain.

Second, unlike glucose, fructose does not stimulate the mechanisms that normally induce satiety, which would signal you to stop eating. Without these appetite-control mechanisms, your appetite has no shutoff signal. You can drink a sixty-four-ounce Big Gulp full of HFCS and your body will not let you know that it is full, or that you've eaten much at all. If you were to eat a similar amount of calories of real food, you would feel stuffed.[24,25] For this reason, many researchers think that the ever-increasing use of HFCS is one of the primary causes of the obesity epidemic.

In the past, fructose was seen as a beneficial sugar for diabetics because it was characterized as only causing a small increase in blood sugar and did not increase insulin. However, given the fact that fructose causes so many health problems, the American Diabetes Association now advises diabetics to avoid refined corn fructose entirely.

The Obesity Epidemic

According to the results of the National Health and Nutrition Examination Survey (NHANES) 1999–2002, an estimated 65 percent of U.S. adults are overweight, with 30 percent of this group classified as obese. The classifications of overweight and obese are based on a person's body mass index (BMI).

BMI	WEIGHT STATUS
Below 18.5	Underweight
18.5–24.9	Normal
25.0–29.9	Overweight
30.0 and up	Obese

Body Mass Index can be calculated using pounds and inches with this equation:

$$BMI = \left[\frac{\text{weight in pounds}}{(\text{height in inches}) \times (\text{height in inches})} \right] \times 703$$

For example, a person who weighs 220 pounds and is 6 feet 3 inches tall has a BMI of 27.5.

$$\frac{220 \text{ lbs.}}{[\ (75 \text{ inches}) \times (75 \text{ inches})\ ]} \times 703 = 27.5$$

In the last twenty years, the obesity rates have doubled. We have also seen the prevalence of overweight children quadruple from 4 percent in 1970 to 16 percent in 2002.[26] The obesity epidemic is also a problem in other industrialized nations, like England, where people subsist on a diet of convenience foods and processed food, and lead sedentary lifestyles similar to those of Americans.

The statistics for diabetes are also daunting. One out of every three U.S. adults—that's 73 million people—have diabetes or its precursor, impaired fasting glucose.[27] Nearly 20 million Americans have full blown diabetes and the other 50+ million have prediabetes. What is really amazing is that one-third of these individuals do not even know they have the disease.[28]

Worldwide the number of people with diabetes is over 200 million. The International Diabetes Foundation predicts this may rise to 333 million people by 2025. In 2005, the World Health Organization warned that deaths from diabetes may increase by 80 percent by 2015.[29]

Sugar and the Environment

In addition to all of the health risks, sugar plantations worldwide have caused widespread destruction by ruining the soil and trees of their surrounding environment. The energy-intensive process of reducing sugarcane to refined sugar has often resulted in the decimation of the local trees as a source for fuel. In tropical areas such as Florida, the Caribbean, Australia, and Hawaii, sediment, pesticides, fertilizer, and liquid wastes from the cane fields are destroying the neighboring swamps, seagrass beds, marine environments, and coral reefs. The book *Bittersweet: The History of Sugar* by Peter Macinnis, from which most of the historical information about sugar in this chapter was obtained, concludes with the following provocative thought: "If we need sweetness in our food, perhaps we should seek other ways of finding it, because right now our joint human sweet tooth looks set to cause a nasty abscess in the environment."[30]

Artificial Sweeteners Are Not the Answer

Americans now consume over twenty pounds of artificial sweeteners per person per year, but it hasn't solved the problem: the rates of weight gain and diabetes and all the other chronic diseases still continue to skyrocket. Not only are artificial sweeteners *not* providing a solution for the obesity epidemic, but these chemicals may be linked to a whole new range of diseases far more harmful than the love handles they were designed to cure. The chemical plants that produce them are even worse for the environment as the sugar plantations. And, just as sugar was once long considered healthy and safe, artificial sweeteners are currently widely regarded as being completely safe and without side effects. For if they caused harm, why would the FDA allow them to be on the market? To answer this question, we will take a detailed look at artificial sweeteners and the operation of the FDA.

CHAPTER TWO:
SWEET NOTHINGS

THE RISE OF THE
ARTIFICIAL SWEETENERS

I would feel more optimistic about a bright future for man if he spent less time proving that he can outwit nature and more time tasting her sweetness and respecting her seniority.
— E. B. White (author of Charlotte's Web *and* Stuart Little)

On a cold February day in 1879, two researchers were experimenting with dangerous chemicals at Johns Hopkins University. Founded only three years previously, Johns Hopkins was America's very first "research" university, not only providing a place for scientists to experiment, but also providing students with an education. And one of its researchers was about to create something unprecedented in human history.

One of the two scientists working in that laboratory was Dr. Ira Remsen, a well-known chemist. He was one of the first five faculty members to be hired there, and he later became the university's president. The other man was Constantine Fahlberg, a research fellow who was working for Remsen. The two were researching toluene derivatives. Toluene is a clear, colorless liquid produced in the process of making gasoline from crude oil, and in making coke (as in carbon residue) from coal. It's used in creating paints, paint thinners, fingernail polish, lacquers, adhesives, and rubber—and it's highly dangerous. The U.S. government's Agency for Toxic Substances and Disease

Registry classifies it as hazardous;[1] exposure to high levels can cause unconsciousness or even death.

But one of these two scientists made a serendipitous discovery while working with a particular chemical made from toluene. He used a method that would soon become a remarkably familiar one in the story of artificial sweeteners: accidentally spilling and then ingesting chemicals. In this particular case, the researcher in question spilled the toluene derivative onto his hand, and later that evening he noticed his food at dinner tasted oddly sweet. He traced the taste back to the chemicals, and named the substance saccharin, after the word *saccharide*, which means complex sugar.[2]

Which man made the discovery? Well, according to Remsen, it was Remsen—but according to Fahlberg, it was Fahlberg. It wasn't much of an issue when the two colleagues jointly published the results of their research in 1879.[3] However, in 1884, Fahlberg patented saccharin and began mass-producing it—without crediting Remsen, Johns Hopkins University, or anyone else. Fahlberg became fabulously wealthy, and Remsen did not. "Fahlberg is a scoundrel," Remsen later commented. "It nauseates me to hear my name mentioned in the same breath with him."[4]

The illustrious history of the marketing of artificial sweeteners had begun.

In fact, the commercialization of saccharin marks something of a turning point in the nature of scientific research. William Brody (a former president of Johns Hopkins, like Remsen) called it "an epochal event in American history . . . you can pretty well pinpoint that moment as the birth of technology transfer, the movement of university-generated research discoveries from abstract ideas to concrete products available on the market and capable of generating a profit."[5] In other words, the date of Fahlberg's patent was the very moment that the pure scientific research of the university system became directly linked to the profit-and-loss margins of industry.

And it therefore also marks the beginning of the era when research needs, scientific funding sources, and, of course, safety concerns could be overpowered or controlled by the desires of the people who were looking to make a quick buck. It's probably not terribly surprising that this period in the history of science starts with a rip-off, a bitter argument, and a lot of money being made by someone.

Saccharin was introduced to the marketplace with great success both in the United States. and Europe. Although the concept of diet foods didn't really exist yet, there was still a brisk business for a substance that was much sweeter per volume than sugar itself.

In fact, the British had a hard time obtaining it for a while, because British law, due to an odd quirk, taxed sweetener based on its sweetening power. Since saccharin was then rated at being five hundred times sweeter than sugar, it was prohibitively expensive—so saccharin was smuggled into the country like an illicit drug.[6]

But such obstacles to saccharin's market power were the exception rather than the rule, as it gradually became a larger and larger industry; in 1901, a company called Monsanto was formed for the sole purpose of producing saccharin. By 1903, Monsanto began producing saccharin for an obscure new company called Coca-Cola. In 1907, saccharin began to be used in products for diabetics, because it did not raise blood sugars.

And in 1912, saccharin was banned as a result of public concerns about possible health risks.

But the ban didn't last very long. In 1914, the sugar rationing of World War I created a demand for artificial sweeteners, and health concerns were brushed aside in the face of economic ones. The war increased the demand for saccharin greatly and turned it into a major product with serious commercial clout. The Second World War had a similar effect, and by 1945 saccharin use was commonplace in the United States and Europe.[7]

> Saccharin contains only one-eighth of a calorie per teaspoon and is approximately three hundred times sweeter than sugar. Saccharin created the foundation for sugar-free products worldwide. It is still used in tabletop sweeteners, toothpaste, baked goods, jams, chewing gum, canned fruit, candy, dessert toppings, salad dressings, and mouthwash. It is stable at high temperatures, so it can be used for cooking, and it is available in both powdered and liquid forms.

Saccharin turned out to be the first of many artificial sweeteners.

What Are Artificial Sweeteners Anyway?

"Artificial" means that the sweetener is not found in nature, but is instead a man-made chemical compound. Artificial sweeteners do not contain

CURRENTLY, THE LIST OF ARTIFICIAL SWEETENERS INCLUDE (IN ORDER OF APPEARANCE):

- Saccharin
- Cyclamate
- Aspartame
- Alitame
- Sucralose
- Acesulfame-K
- Neotame

nutrients like vitamins and minerals, and they are very low in carbohydrates and calories. They are appealing because they provide a sweet taste without the calories or consequences of eating sugar (which contains fifteen calories per teaspoon).

My position on all artificial sweeteners is that you should simply avoid them: I believe that you should stick to the food your body was designed to eat, ideally foods as they are found in their unprocessed state in nature. Nevertheless, if you choose to use one or more of these sweeteners, some are better than others in terms of safety—and it's useful to know a bit about their history in order to assess the risk.

Saccharin and Cyclamate are Not as Dangerous

It might surprise you to know that saccharin, with its carcinogenic reputation, and cyclamate, which is still banned in the United States, are probably among the less risky artificial sweeteners (although I still do not recommended them).

It might also surprise you to learn that the long-term risks of common sweeteners like Splenda are unknown. In fact, history shows us that which sweeteners are approved for public use and which are not generally has little to do with public health, and everything to do with which corporations have enough influence in the FDA.

The Sweetener Cycle

The history of the sweeteners discussed in this book all follow, with minor variations, a similar and disturbing pattern: A scientist accidentally discovers that a chemical he is experimenting with tastes sweet. A manufacturer buys the patented chemical and convinces the FDA to approve it—often without adequate research or long-term studies. Then the sweetener enters the marketplace with a great deal of ballyhoo, and the manufacturers of diet products scramble to add the new sweetener to their products to catch the wave of media exposure. The public eagerly embraces the new sweetener, and the consumption dramatically increases.

Over the years, complaints to the FDA regarding the sweetener start to accumulate, as some people become ill from its long-term use. The side effects that people experience spur an investigation, and researchers examine previous studies or conduct new ones to uncover the health risks that may have been unidentified, suppressed, or ignored. The sweetener may or may not be removed from the market, but it is of little consequence because suddenly a new sweetener is introduced to the market to replace it, and everyone flocks to the new artificial sweetener promised land, hoping that there won't be any harmful consequences with the new one—the current stage in the life cycle of Splenda.

Cyclamate—the next popular artificial sweetener to be created after saccharin—followed this pattern fairly closely, although with some interesting twists.

Cyclamate: Questionable Studies and Questionable Actions

In 1937, University of Illinois graduate student Michael Sveda discovered cyclamate using a method astonishingly similar to the one used to find saccharin nearly sixty years previously. Sveda was trying to synthesize antipyretic (fever-reducing) drugs in the laboratory and laid the cigarette he was smoking down on a lab bench. When he placed it in his mouth again, he discovered the sweet taste of cyclamate from the antipyretic drugs he had on his fingers.

Cyclamate had not been the very next sweetener to be artificially created after saccharin. Dulcin, for example, was developed only a few years after saccharin by J. Berlinerbrau, and was occasionally used in the early twentieth century—until a long-term study finally done in the 1950s demonstrated that it was toxic for sustained use even at small doses. But cyclamate was, however, the first artificial sweetener after saccharin to achieve (and aid) saccharin's widespread commercial popularity.

Cyclamate had less aftertaste than saccharin, was soluble in water, was stable when heated, was inexpensive to produce, and contained zero calories.

Dupont produced the first patent for cyclamate and later sold it to Abbott Laboratories. Abbott submitted a "New Drug Application" to the FDA for cyclamate in 1950; they wanted to use it to mask the bitter taste of their new pharmaceutical products.

Both saccharin and cyclamate were introduced before the Food Additives Amendment to the Food, Drug, and Cosmetic Act, which you'll read more about in chapter 5. Both were therefore automatically classified in the Generally Recognized As Safe (GRAS) food additive category when the act was passed in 1958, meaning neither was required to be thoroughly tested using studies designed for safety analyses.

Cyclamate was recommended for diabetics as a tabletop sweetener. The result was the introduction of the very first powdered artificial sweetener blend—Sweet'N Low®, manufactured by Cumberland Packing Corp.

Sweet'N Low originally was a mixture of cyclamate and saccharin in a ten-to-one ratio; the mixture masks the off-taste of each sweetener, particularly the somewhat metallic aftertaste of saccharin. In addition to being the first blend of artificial sweeteners, it was also the first artificial sweetening agent to be marketed in powdered form, imitating the appearance, texture, and taste of sugar.

It was a tremendous commercial success, and to this day, little pink packets of Sweet'N Low are a familiar sight at restaurants and coffee shops across the United States. Along with Sweet'N Low, diet drinks such as Diet Rite (Royal Crown Cola—1958) and Tab (Coca-Cola Co.—1963) were also introduced, using the same cyclamate/saccharin blend with great financial success.

But in 1969, cyclamate was suddenly banned by the FDA. New research studies seemed to indicate that cyclamate caused cancer in laboratory mice.[8] The FDA banned cyclamate right away; one part of the 1958 Food Additives Amendment, the Delaney Clause, sets a zero tolerance for any chemical found to cause cancer in animal testing.

However, certain details do seem to raise questions as to whether the FDA was acting out of concern for the well-being of the public or concern for the well-being of a competing manufacturer. It's an interesting coincidence, for example, that 1969 was also the year that G. D. Searle, the manufacturer of aspartame (NutraSweet) first applied for an FDA patent, just a few years after it had been discovered (by way of an accidental spill of chemicals onto chemist James M. Schlatter's finger, which he then licked).

The scientific study that caused the cyclamate ban did show the chemical caused bladder tumors in rats and mice—when they were given a dosage equal to a human drinking ten gallons per day for a year of a cyclamate-sweetened drink. Most other countries never acted on the questionable studies; cyclamate continues to be used in more than fifty-five countries including the British Commonwealth.

But once cyclamate was taken off the market, Abbott Labs held the burden of proof for showing that it was safe before it could be marketed again. Abbott has persistently submitted additional safety data, sent petitions, and requested hearings from the FDA in a vain effort to get cyclamate re-approved. In 1973, Abbott submitted a petition to gain approval for cyclamates as a new food additive, which placed the FDA under tremendous scrutiny by all interested parties. The agency had to consider whether to reverse its previous decision while still assuring the public that the safety standard had been met. The major concerns to the regulatory scientific reviewers were experiments in rats and dogs that showed cyclohexylamine, a metabolite of cyclamate, caused testicular atrophy and reduced sperm production.[9-12] Other studies showed adverse effects such as bladder tumors and cardiotoxicity. Abbott countered that they were not able to replicate the results in their own studies and therefore cyclamate was safe.

There were several rounds of scientific review and debate about incomplete data and interpretation of data. The controversy over the potential health hazards of cyclamate has continued for over thirty years. Some issues were resolved, while others remained as major scientific safety concerns. Both Abbott Laboratories and the FDA have poured significant resources into the cyclamate review process.

One major obstacle to the FDA approval of cyclamate is its relatively low Acceptable Daily Intake (ADI) of about 200 to 300 mg per day for the average 60 kg adult (and proportionally less for children). Based on current artificial sweetener use, approval of cyclamate for general use would result in consumers exceeding the ADI. Therefore, if the FDA approves cyclamate, it would be sanctioning a product likely to be consumed beyond the safe conditions of use. The FDA has also argued that it has also never been demonstrated that cyclamate does not cause cancer in humans or animals, and is not a mutagen.

However, in 1985, the Cancer Assessment Committee of FDA's Center for Food Safety and Applied Nutrition concluded that cyclamate is not a carcinogen. At the FDA's request, the National Academy of Sciences conducted a comprehensive review and also concluded that cyclamate does not cause cancer.[13]

The FDA still has not approved cyclamate.

When you read the chapter on aspartame, you'll notice a distinct difference in the FDA's treatment of the two chemicals. After the ban on cyclamate went into effect, aspartame was approved by the FDA in spite of copious evidence of adverse effects—far more, in fact, than cyclamate has ever been accused of. It seems somewhat arbitrary . . . or it makes you wonder just who's really making the critical decisions at the FDA.

Sweet'N Low is currently a mixture of saccharin and dextrose. You'll find out more about aspartame in chapter 3, and more about the FDA approval process in chapter 5.

"Saccharin Has Been Determined to Cause Cancer in Laboratory Animals"

The concern over cyclamate and cancer after the 1969 studies resulted in saccharin being tested for safety for the very first time—nearly one hundred years after its introduction into the human diet. In the late 1970s, a scientist in Canada named Douglas Arnold performed a study finding that saccharin caused bladder cancer in 50 percent of the laboratory animals fed high doses of saccharin (although this has not been shown in humans). Additional studies confirmed the increased risk of bladder tumors in animals.[14–16]

The Canadian government immediately outlawed saccharin. Influenced by the actions of Canada, the FDA began its own research regarding saccharin safety and proposed to likewise ban the sweetener under the terms of the anticarcinogen protections in the Delaney Clause just as they did with cyclamate. As I mentioned earlier, the Delaney Clause sets a zero tolerance for any chemical found to cause cancer in animal testing. This was met by a great deal of public opposition, as saccharin was at that time the only artificial sweetener available for general use; cyclamate was, of course, already off the market, and aspartame had only been approved for limited usage. Congress intervened and allowed saccharin to be sold as long as the products containing it carried a warning label reading: "Use of this product may be hazardous to your health. This product contains saccharin, which has been determined to cause cancer in laboratory animals."[17]

The FDA rescinded their proposal to ban saccharin in 1991 due to the results of long-term studies that had been conducted on people with high saccharin use. These studies, mostly on diabetics, did demonstrate some correlation between saccharin use and cancer, but not enough for saccharin to be considered a major cancer risk factor. Moreover, in 1992, tests performed on rats showed that they had physiological differences from humans that made them more susceptible to bladder cancer from saccharin. So in 2000, President Clinton signed into law that the cancer warnings were no longer required for saccharin products.[18]

However, all of that should still have been irrelevant based on the Delaney Clause, which was put into place to avoid unnecessary carcinogens in the food supply. Under the law, if it causes cancer in animals, it's supposed to be banned.[19] Instead, Congress removed even the requirement of placing a warning label on saccharin-containing products. Apparently, the FDA's opinion is that if saccharin is not a *major risk factor*, but merely a *risk factor*, the product should be available and the public deserves no warning.

Nonetheless, somewhat ironically considering its reputation, saccharin is probably the safest artificial sweetener on the market. But considering it has a bitter aftertaste, is derived from toluene, and is not a natural food, I believe even it should be avoided.

Aspartame, Alitame, Sucralose

In spite of the concerns about saccharin and cyclamate, the growing diet-food industry fueled an ever-increasing demand for artificial sweeteners over the decades that followed—and now the world consumption of artificial sweeteners stands at 7.5 million metric tons per year. Looking only at diet sodas, over four billion gallons per year are now being sold, and they account for an ever-increasing share of the vast soft-drink market. As noncaloric sweetening has become a progressively larger business, increasing revenues have been earmarked for finding and developing new varieties of usable chemicals.

The next three major artificial sweeteners to be introduced after cyclamate were aspartame, alitame, and sucralose. Knowledge of the potentially hazardous effects of these "second-generation" sweeteners is limited to the toxicological animal data that is required for FDA approval. There are no large-scale human studies that investigate potential risks for birth defects, DNA damage, or cancer for the newer sweeteners. It's too early to establish their impact on people who consume them regularly, especially since the sweeteners are often mixed together, and there is absolutely no animal, human, or even in vitro evidence that any combination of several artificial sweeteners is safe to consume.

Aspartame was the first artificial sweetener to fall under the 1958 amendments requiring premarket proof of safety. The approval of aspartame, and its safety record since, are important enough that the entire next chapter of this book has been devoted to it. Sucralose (Splenda)—the most popular artificial sweetener currently available—also merits a more in-depth look, so we will cover it more thoroughly in chapter 4. Sucralose, incidentally, was discovered when a graduate student misunderstood a request for "testing" of a chemical as a request for "tasting" it.[20]

Alitame (brand name Aclame™) was developed in 1979; it was the result of intensive research that started in the early 1970s at the pharmaceutical company Pfizer Inc. after the discovery of aspartame showed the potential of dipeptides as high-intensity sweeteners. Alitame is made from the amino acids L-aspartic acid and D-alanine, and a tetramethylthietanyl-amine moiety. Pfizer has conducted animal and human studies to support the safety of alitame. The petition for regulatory

> Alitame is a white crystalline powder with a faint alcohol odor. It's soluble in water and heat stable. Alitame is already approved for use in a variety of food and beverage products in Australia, New Zealand, Mexico, and China. Safety studies so far have not shown it to cause cancer, but alitame is a closely related cousin of aspartame, sharing many of its characteristics, and therefore you should read chapter 3 on aspartame to make an informed choice about compounds of this nature.

approval in the United States was submitted in 1986 and is still under consideration.

Approximately fifteen studies have been submitted to the FDA to prove alitame's safety, but the FDA has requested that one questionable animal study be repeated. This additional study is expected to delay alitame's approval in the United States.

For the time being, little is known about alitame. Advocates for its approval describe one of alitame's main assets as being its synergistic sweetening effect when combined with other low-calorie sweeteners. So it would seem prudent, if the goal is to use alitame as a synergistic sweetener, that it be tested for safety in combination with other artificial sweeteners, but this is unlikely to happen.

Acesulfame-K (Ace-K, Sunett®)

Sunett is the brand name and registered trademark for the sweetener acesulfame potassium, or acesulfame-K, which is manufactured by Nutrinova. It is composed of carbon, nitrogen, oxygen, hydrogen, sulfur, and potassium. Those same elements are also found in fertilizer. And it was discovered in 1967 when chemist Karl Clauss, of the Hoechst AG Company, accidentally spilled some on his finger, which he then licked as he reached for a piece of paper.

Acesulfame-K was first approved for limited use by the FDA in July 1988, and then additionally approved for use in beverages in 1998, although European countries had been using acesulfame-K for over fifteen years prior to U.S. approval. PepsiCo was the first soft-drink company to use acesulfame-K in their new Pepsi ONE® soda, but it is now used in many brands of sodas, fruit drinks, and nutraceutical beverages in the United States.

The details of acesulfame-K's road to approval are not widely publicized. In 1988, aspartame was capturing both positive and negative public attention, while acesulfame-K quietly earned limited approval for use in chewing gum, sugar-free baked goods, and gelatin desserts.[21-23]

The notable advantage of acesulfame-K is that it acts as a flavor enhancer and preserves the sweetness of sweet foods. It is also heat stable, so it can be used in baking. But its safety has been questioned.

In the mid-1990s, Hoechst petitioned the FDA for acesulfame-K to be approved for use in soft drinks, which greatly increases consumer exposure. It was at this point that concerned scientists raised objections. Numerous prominent U.S. scientists opposed introduction of acesulfame-K as a non-nutritive beverage sweetener, including Dr. David Rall, former director of the National Institute of Environmental Sciences; Dr. Arthur Upton, former director of the National Cancer Institute; and Dr. Umberto Saffiotti, chief of the National Cancer Institute's laboratory of experimental pathology.

They asserted that the studies on which the sweetener's existing approval was based were seriously flawed, and that wider approval would lead to a public danger. Dr. Saffiotti pointed out that the original studies of acesulfame-K were done in the 1970s, when "the standard criteria for the design of animal carcinogenesis bioassays were still under development."[24]

The Center for Science in the Public Interest (CSPI)—a nonprofit agency to protect the public—has repeatedly expressed concern that acesulfame-K is a potential carcinogen.[25]

In June 1995, CSPI filed a protest with the FDA, saying that the sweetener's carcinogenicity had not been properly tested in long-term animal feeding tests. CSPI strongly urged that the FDA require further testing before permitting acesulfame-K to be permitted in soft drinks.

The book *Safe Food*, by Dr. Michael Jacobson and other CSPI researchers, describes the sweetener as follows:

> The public is waiting for an artificial sweetener that is unquestionably safe. But this one isn't it. Even compared to aspartame and saccharin . . . acesulfame-K is the worst. The additive is inadequately tested; the FDA based its approval on tests of acesulfame-K that fell short of the FDA's own standards. But even those tests indicate that the additive causes cancer in animals, which means it may increase cancer risk in humans.[26]

Acesulfame-K may, among other problems, contain methylene chloride, a known carcinogen. The FDA Final Report 59 FR 61538 on acesulfame-K, dated December 1, 1994, admits:

> Methylene chloride, a carcinogenic chemical, is a potential impurity in acesulfame-K resulting from its use as a solvent in the initial manufacturing step of the sweetener.

The Material Safety Data Sheets concerning methylene chloride warn that chronic exposure can cause headaches, mental confusion, depression, liver effects, kidney effects, bronchitis, loss of appetite, nausea, lack of balance, visual disturbances, and *cancer in humans.*[27]

The FDA acknowledged that the initial testing conducted by Hoechst was less than adequate. However, the agency stated that they had asked the company to perform additional tests, which they then found acceptable.[28] Regardless of the validity of the studies submitted by Hoechst, the FDA had an ulterior motive to approve the expanded use of acesulfame-K; if the FDA were to delay its approval of acesulfame-K for use in diet soda, they would be admitting to not adequately assessing its safety during its initial approval.

Scientific opposition to acesulfame-K has been ignored. The FDA has not required any further safety testing to address the legitimate scientific concerns raised by CSPI. Instead, the FDA has now increased consumer exposure even further by approving its broader use in baked goods, yogurts, and some alcoholic drinks such as wine coolers.

The end result is that we now have another sweetener that has not undergone the rigid safety testing that would validate its widespread use.

Neotame

In 1985, the chemical giant Monsanto acquired aspartame from G. D. Searle and established a separate subsidiary named the NutraSweet Company. As the patent for aspartame was running out, Monsanto developed a new version of aspartame called neotame that is seventy-two times sweeter. Neotame is chemically related to aspartame, but has greater heat stability, which is an attractive quality for use in baked goods.

Neotame was approved in 1997 for tabletop sweetener use, and in 2002 as a general-use sweetener. The sweetest artificial sweetener ever invented, neotame is seven to thirteen thousand times the sweetness of sugar. Neotame is *aspartame* plus 3-di-methyl-butyl, which can be found on the EPA's list of most hazardous chemicals. Unlike aspartame, neotame is not broken down in your body into the amino acid phenylalanine, which is toxic to people with the rare disorder phenylketonuria (PKU).

For some reason, neotame has not been launched with the massive marketing campaign of its cousin aspartame; it seems as if the food manufacturers are being discreet about adding neotame to their products. We found it very difficult to even find a list of products that contained neotame. The official Web site, www.neotame.com, is relatively devoid of useful information, and they have not responded to our multiple requests for information. According to Food Navigator-USA, sales of neotame increased by 400 percent from 2004 to 2005. Some of the new products containing neotame include the grocery store chain Kroger's fruit juice and certain iced-tea powders, Detour energy bars, Wrigley Chewing Gum in Australia, Roman Meal Bread line, and Herr's pretzels in the United States.[29]

Prior to approval, consumer advocacy groups submitted comments objecting to neotame. Objections centered on the similarities between neotame and aspartame; since the chemical structure is similar to aspartame, it is logical to assume that some of the same toxicity concerns that exist for aspartame will apply. Just like its chemical cousin, neotame contains aspartic acid, which caused "holes in the brains" of lab animals, and methanol, which is capable of causing blindness, liver damage, and death (you'll learn about all of these dangers in detail in the next chapter). Despite these problems, neotame was approved and is considered safe for people of all ages, including pregnant or breastfeeding women, teens, and children.

According to Neotame.com, neotame is a flavor enhancer having the ability to "bring flavors to life." The Web site also reports, "Over 100 scientific studies were done to establish the safety of neotame. A comprehensive battery of safety studies in animals and humans demonstrated no adverse effects from neotame."[30]

Our preliminary analysis of neotame research does not, in our opinion, prove that neotame is safe. As of July 2006 only nineteen studies were indexed in the National Library of Medicine, and half of those studies had absolutely nothing to do with safety. Two articles addressed weight changes in rats, and one examined blood sugar control, but there were no articles that directly studied the neurotoxicity, immunology, development, and safety of neotame, nor were there any long-term studies on humans.

The remaining 80 percent of studies that Monsanto references were unpublished internal studies funded by Monsanto. So none of the safety studies were done by an independent lab. As you will see in the next chapter, this is most concerning considering the notorious conflicts of interests that emerged in the independent and manufacturer funded studies of aspartame.

When Monsanto applied for FDA approval for neotame in 1998, the nonprofit group Truth in Labeling requested a copy of the application under the Freedom of Information Act. The FDA said that they would not send them the information and that they would have to come to FDA headquarters if they wanted to see it. According to Jack Samuels of Truth in Labeling,

> We went to Washington, DC, and did review the file on a very hot day, in a small room that had no windows or air conditioning. FDA staff checked on us every few minutes. At the time of our review of Monsanto's application, three human studies on the safety of Neotame were presented. The studies had few subjects, all of whom were employees of the company. Some of the subjects reported headaches after ingesting Neotame, but the researcher concluded that the headaches were not related to Neotame ingestion. Not mentioned in the studies was the fact that migraine headache is, by far, the most commonly reported adverse reaction to aspartame in the files of the FDA. The FDA has over 7,000 reports of adverse reactions to aspartame. The reported reactions include death.[31]

Blended Artificial Sweeteners

With the variety of artificial sweeteners now available, many are now combined in sweetener blends—the mixing of multiple sweeteners together, first seen in Sweet'N Low. Blends combine sweeteners such as sucralose, aspartame, acesulfame-K, sorbitol, xylitol, high-fructose corn syrup (HFCS), and even cyclamate (in Canada and Europe). Acesulfame-K and Splenda are now the top two artificial sweeteners used in blends.

Sweetener blends are now the norm in the diet industry because of their three key advantages:

- **Cost savings.** The combination of artificial sweeteners can be sweeter than either artificial sweetener alone, requiring smaller amounts of each chemical. For example, acesulfame-K is even sweeter when used in combination with aspartame, the combination used in the one-calorie drink Pepsi ONE. Blending a more expensive sweetener with a less expensive one also saves money.

- **Taste.** A blend can disguise an individual sweetener's unappealing flavor (like that of aspartame), such as in the case of C2 Coke®, which uses a blend of aspartame and HFCS to produce a drink that tastes as much like the original beverage as possible, but which has half the calories.

- **Flexibility.** Blending sweeteners allows for more options for new products. Consumers can choose between the no-calorie products or the reduced-calorie products containing a blend of HFCS with artificial sweeteners.

Many soft-drink companies are currently marketing "mid-calorie" sodas that have 50 percent HFCS and 50 percent sweetener blends. This type of soda is targeting consumers who dislike the chemical taste in diet sodas but still feel guilty about the sugar in regular sodas. C2 Coke is a prime example of these types of sodas and is advertised as having half the carbs, half the calories, and half the sugar of regular Coca-Cola.

The diet-food industry is not the only one mixing the artificial sweeteners. People do that too. Some may choose to have Splenda in their coffee at home in the morning, but the coffee shop near work only has Sweet'N Low—so that's what gets used in the afternoon. Then they chew sugar-free gum periodically throughout the day, which contains a third sweetener, perhaps aspartame. A Diet Pepsi™ with lunch adds a chemical cocktail of aspartame and acesulfame-K.

The combination of artificial sweeteners presents a vast array of potential problems. We have a long history of monitoring drug use that has allowed us to appreciate that there is an exponential increase in side effects that is directly proportional to the number of drugs one is taking. There is a similar potential harm from the interactions of artificial sweetener combinations in the body.

Combining these chemicals begs a few questions:

- Will the combination have a synergistic effect and result in a more toxic compound than either one alone?

- How will the interaction of the *chemicals* affect your body?

- How will the interaction of the *breakdown products* affect your body?

There are no research studies being conducted to answer these questions—so we will simply have to wait and watch for symptoms in the human guinea pigs who choose to consume these chemical cocktails over time.

The Next Big Thing?

Right now, Splenda is the blockbuster new artificial sweetener, with millions of users. However, people are still wary from the disconcerting history of previous artificial sweeteners, and thousands of people every day are searching "Splenda" on Google or Mercola.com to determine if it is as safe as the manufacturer claims it is. But because there are no long-term studies on Splenda, we will have to wait to see the results of people using it over an extended period of time.

Hopefully the material presented in this book will cause you to seriously revise your understanding about the safety of consuming these common artificial sweeteners. Some of you love to drink diet soda and some of you add Equal® to your coffee every day. Before you take another sip, sit down to read this next chapter on aspartame.

CHAPTER THREE: SWEET AGONY

THE SHOCKING STORY OF ASPARTAME

PETER'S STORY

Peter was driving to work on the highway when his vision suddenly flipped 180 degrees.

Everything was upside down. The other cars were still in their lanes, but they looked like they were driving on the ceiling. Where his brain was telling him the ground should be was nothing but a dizzying expanse of sky.

Peter managed to hit the emergency blinkers on his dashboard and somehow maneuvered his upside-down car over to the shoulder in the center divide. An ambulance took him to the emergency room.

At the emergency room doctors ran numerous tests, but they all came back negative. All the while, Peter's vision remained bizarrely inverted. After three hours, the ER doctor asked Peter a strange question: had Peter been drinking any diet sodas?

Peter responded that, yes, he'd been drinking two Diet Pepsi's per day for the past two weeks—he was on a diet and trying to lose twenty pounds.

The doctor responded that the vision problem was probably a direct result of the aspartame found in many diet sodas, and had been traced as the cause in the majority of patients seen in the ER with symptoms similar to Peter's.

Peter's vision returned to normal about half an hour later. But he doesn't drink diet soda anymore.

History of Aspartame

Aspartame, discovered in 1965, was a product of the first generation of artificial sweeteners. It was the third artificial sweetener identified to achieve acceptance in the general market, and it dominated the industry until Splenda came along in the late nineties. You may recognize aspartame by its other names: NutraSweet and Equal. Equal is more easily recognized as the little blue packets found on nearly every restaurant table in the United States.

Today, NutraSweet is sold in over one hundred countries, found in over six thousand products, and is consumed by over 250 million people. It's found in most diet sodas and a good portion of chewing gum. In fact, many find it difficult to actually find chewing gum in their local grocery store that doesn't contain aspartame. To place its success in perspective, over two-thirds of the U.S. population currently use the many thousands of diet sodas and products—including an ever-expanding list of new diet and low-carb consumer goods that may have a great potential for adverse health effects.

The head of Searle's NutraSweet Division, Robert Shapiro, said in 1984 that aspartame was the most thoroughly tested food additive in history.[1] But as you will discover in this chapter, aspartame has had anything but a scientifically valid road to financial success. Its approval process was linked with scandal and coercion within the FDA, the pharmaceutical industry, and other big businesses in corporate America.

H. J. Roberts, MD, coined the term "aspartame disease" to encompass the symptoms, complications, public health implications, and medicolegal ramifications of this chemical sweetener. He has written a massive 1,038-page medical text called *Aspartame Disease: An Ignored Epidemic* addressing the many types of health problems that can occur from aspartame use.[2] There have been more reports to the FDA for aspartame reactions than all other food additives combined (with the exception of Olestra®). Dr. Roberts states that by 1988, *80 percent of complaints to the FDA about food additives* had to deal with aspartame products.[3]

Unlike some of the new sweeteners, such as Splenda, that claim to have little metabolization (broken down) in the body, aspartame is completely metabolized, and the by-products, such as methanol, can cause major complications. Aspartame is undoubtedly one of the most controversial food additives in modern times.

Oops, I Did It Again

As was mentioned in the last chapter, aspartame, like most other artificial sweeteners, was discovered accidentally. Aspartame was originally developed in a laboratory as a drug to treat peptic ulcer disease. In 1965, James Schlatter, a scientist at G. D. Searle & Company, was working on research dealing with amino acids. When he licked his fingers to pick up a piece of paper, Schlatter got the world's first taste of aspartame. As a result, his amino acid combination never found its way to the pharmaceutical industry as a drug. Instead he revolutionized the artificial sweetener industry, never to be the same again.

Early Safety Studies Showing
Brain Damage Were Buried

Senior FDA scientists and consultants vigorously protested approving the release of aspartame products. Their objections were related to the following:

- Disturbing findings in animal studies (especially the frequency of brain tumors)

- Seemingly flawed experimental data

- The absence of extensive premarketing trials on humans using actual products containing aspartame over prolonged periods

Early safety studies of aspartame conducted in 1967 by Harold Waisman for G. D. Searle & Company identified potential neurotoxic side effects. In one study, out of seven monkeys fed aspartame mixed with milk, one monkey actually died, and five others had grand mal seizures. Other studies performed by neuroscientist Dr. John Olney showed that aspartic acid, one of the main ingredients in aspartame, caused damage to the brains of infant mice. Searle's own scientists confirmed these findings in a similar study.[4]

Aspartame Replaces Cyclamates and Saccharin

Despite early evidence of neurotoxicity, executives at G. D. Searle had incentive to push forward with their new compound. As you'll recall, during the early 1970s cyclamate was pulled off the market because of cancer concerns. All the while, scientists were seriously questioning the safety of saccharin. The media was denouncing the only two available artificial sweeteners, and the time was ripe for their replacement.

Corporate leaders at G. D. Searle, realizing that the market was wide open for a new sugar substitute, decided to invest tens of millions of dollars into conducting the necessary tests for aspartame's approval. In addition, Searle executives developed a political strategy aimed at ensuring that the FDA's view of aspartame would be a positive one.[5,6]

In February 1973, the Searle Company submitted an application that included over one hundred studies to the FDA. Later that year the FDA ruled that the information Searle provided was inadequate to determine aspartame's safety. The FDA requested further testing, and after receiving the information in July 1974, aspartame was granted preliminary approval for restricted use.

Aspartame Safety Data Seriously Flawed—
and Causes First Ever FDA-Initiated
Criminal Investigation

The safety and the validity of Searle's aspartame data was immediately challenged. A petition initiated by attorney Jim Turner and Dr. John Olney triggered the FDA to investigate the laboratory practices of G. D. Searle's scientists. These investigations led to serious questions about the accuracy of the studies they submitted and delayed the final approval of aspartame.

In 1977, the FDA requested the U.S. attorney's office to investigate Searle for alleged inaccuracies and inadequate testing procedures for their aspartame studies and for misrepresenting their findings[7]—the first time in history that the FDA requested a criminal investigation of a food manufacturer. Searle was investigated for knowingly misrepresenting their findings from safety tests on aspartame. While investigating potential deliberate criminal acts, the probe into Searle's activities uncovered many inaccuracies and inadequate testing procedures used in their aspartame studies.[8, 9]

Searle Avoids Federal Indictment

At the very same time in 1977 that the grand jury was investigating Searle's activities, the law firm that represented Searle began contract negotiations with Samuel Skinner—the U.S. attorney leading the investigation. In July 1977, Skinner left the U.S. attorney's office and took a position with the Searle's law firm, Sidley & Austin. Skinner's sudden resignation stalled the grand jury investigation for long enough that the statute of limitations ran out. As a result, the grand jury was forced to effectively abandon its investigation. In my view, Skinner's reprehensible actions deserved punishment of the highest order. In fact he was rewarded throughout his career with other prominent government positions, such as secretary of transportation and chief of staff for President H. W. Bush.

In August of 1977, the FDA released the Bressler Report, by Dr. Jerome Bressler, which identified additional errors and inconsistent findings in the aspartame safety studies.

In 1979, the FDA established a Public Board of Inquiry (PBOI) to rule on safety issues surrounding NutraSweet and within one year concluded that aspartame should not be approved pending further investigations of brain tumors in animals. The board determined that it had not been presented with proof of reasonable certainty that aspartame is safe for use as a food additive. Their main concern surrounded the potential risk of increased brain tumors found in animal studies.

The Bressler Report Criticizes Searle Studies

The most controversial aspect of the G. D. Searle studies of rats was revealed in the Bressler Report. The Bressler Report was extremely critical of Searle's studies, because it detailed how Searle had numerous errors and inconsistencies between the original observations on the pathology sheets and the observations submitted to the FDA. He found that animals died after being fed aspartame, and that their autopsies were not done immediately. In fact, some of the autopsies were not performed until one year after the animal's death. By this time, tissues had begun to break down and liquefy, virtually destroying any ability to obtain accurate data.[10] According to Dr. Betty Martini of Dorway.com—a nonprofit Web site dedicated to warning people about aspartame toxicity—Jerome Bressler said that Searle's research was the worst research he had ever seen in his professional experience and that the FDA deleted the worst 20 percent of his findings from the report. Dr. Bressler's doctored report can be viewed at www.dorway.com/bressler.txt.

They also reported obvious tumors as normal—in one case an enlarged lymph node, which was determined to be malignant lymphoma, was recorded as being "normal lymphatic swelling." They covered up a tremendous amount of data that was obviously anything but normal.[11]

Donald Rumsfeld Gets Aspartame Approved

The negative results reported in the Bressler Report were not winning points with the FDA scientific approval process. Therefore, Searle executives decided that they needed a new strategy that would shift focus toward the political approval of aspartame.[12] In March of 1977, political powerhouse Donald Rumsfeld, who would later become the U.S. secretary of defense in the George W. Bush administration, joined G. D. Searle as the new CEO. Rumsfeld quickly brought in several additional political moguls into Searle's top management.[13]

In 1981, Rumsfeld, as CEO of Searle, reportedly made a commitment to getting aspartame approved within a year. He stated that he would use his political influence within Washington to expedite approval.[14] What gave Rumsfeld his confidence was that Rumsfeld's political ally, Ronald Reagan, had just become the fortieth president of the United States. The first thing Reagan did in office was issue an executive order that would limit the power of the current FDA commissioner so that he could not unilaterally prevent aspartame from being approved. Within one month Reagan replaced the commissioner with his puppet, Dr. Arthur Hull Hayes.[15]

Massive Conflict of Interest

Dr. Hayes then appointed an internal panel to review the issues raised by the 1980 FDA Public Board of Inquiry. Three of the five in-house FDA scientists who were responsible for reviewing the brain tumor issues, Dr. Robert Condon, Dr. Satya Dubey, and Dr. Douglas Park, advised against approval of aspartame, stating on the record that the Searle tests are unreliable and not adequate to determine the safety of aspartame.[16]

After the panel ruled three-to-two to uphold the ban for aspartame approval, Dr. Hayes installed a sixth member who tied the vote, which allowed him to cast another vote to break the tie and approve aspartame.[17]

Dr. Hayes had virtually no background in food additives and ignored the recommendations of his own internal FDA team. He immediately took a job with G. D. Searle's public relations firm as a senior scientific consultant and was reportedly paid $1,000 a day.[18,19]

Despite the countless unresolved safety concerns, aspartame plowed ahead. Within one year of aspartame's approval for dry products, G. D. Searle petitioned to allow aspartame to be added to carbonated beverages. The National Soft Drink Association officially objected to this petition because of aspartame's heat instability in liquid form, degrading to diketopiperazine (DKP), methanol, aspartic acid, and phenylalanine. The FDA responded that it was aware that temperature may affect carbonated liquids containing aspartame but that proper shipping and marketing procedures should solve that problem.[20] The problem was not solved. Analyses showed that in beverages stored for eight weeks at room temperature, the amount of aspartame had decreased between 11 and 16 percent. In spite of this, aspartame was approved for use in carbonated beverages in July of 1983.[21]

Consumer Complaints Regarding
Aspartame Side Effects

Less than one year after the first carbonated beverages containing aspartame hit the market, the FDA had almost six hundred consumer complaints regarding aspartame's side effects. Headaches, dizziness, and other reactions filled the FDA files, which forced the FDA to have the Centers for Disease Control (CDC) look into the complaints. The CDC reviewed 213 of 592 cases of aspartame complaints. The reported symptoms included aggressive behavior, disorientation, hyperactivity, extreme numbness, excitability, memory loss, loss of depth perception, liver impairment, cardiac arrest, seizures, suicidal tendencies, severe mood swings, and death. The CDC stated in its 146-page report that further investigation into the neurological and behavioral problems triggered by aspartame was needed. Frederick Trowbridge of the CDC added a sugar-coated executive summary to the CDC report, which is what you will receive if you request the report from the CDC:

> Currently available information, based on data with limitations as described in the report indicated a wide variety of complaints that are generally of a mild nature. Although it may be that certain individuals have an unusual sensitivity to the product, these data do not provide evidence for the existence of serious, widespread, adverse health consequences to the use of aspartame.

The report details case studies of people struggling with serious symptoms for months before they stopped aspartame and their symptoms disappeared. Most of the case reports are not complaints of a "mild nature" as Trowbridge states. I wonder if he even read the report when he wrote the summary. Read the real report for yourself at www.dorway.com/cdctext.txt and see if you come to the same conclusion.[22,23]

Who Is Funding the Studies?

It's important to understand that the source of funds for a study strongly influences the conclusion and findings. This becomes crystal clear when you examine the results of aspartame research.

In an analysis of 166 articles published in medical journals from 1980 to 1985, Dr. Ralph G. Walton, a professor of psychiatry at Northeastern Ohio Universities College of Medicine, found that 100 percent of the seventy-four studies financed by the industry attested to the sweetener's safety. However, of the ninety-two independently funded articles, 91 percent identified adverse health effects.[24] This point was more recently confirmed in research out of Harvard that demonstrated a similar pattern supporting the use of drugs in studies that were funded by the drug company relative to those that were funded by independent organizations.[25]

This is an absolutely amazing contrast. You could predict with a high degree of certainty the results of the study before it was completed by merely finding out who funded the research.

When you look at the history of aspartame's approval, it appears that the industry-supported data was manipulated, or in some cases simply suppressed. The flaws in the studies included:

- Improper protocols

- Omission of critical data

- The use of aspartame in its raw form, rather than in products such as diet sodas or yogurt

One of the problems with the scientific studies conducted on artificial sweeteners, aspartame in particular, is that the clinical trials used the artificial sweetener in its pure powder form. No consumer will ever ingest aspartame in this ideal, pure form; nearly all of the aspartame will be modified by the foods it is mixed with and stored with. There simply are no studies that evaluate aspartame in the form it is typically encountered in the consumer market. For example, there are no studies to evaluate the aspartame breakdown products in diet sodas that may have been sitting in the back of a hot truck, then on a shelf for months. In the case of aspartame, and many other food additives, the unstable conditions frequently encountered can increase breakdown products, which can also significantly increase their injurious effects.[26]

In summary, the safety of aspartame was based on a series of studies completed by its own manufacturers in the 1960s and '70s. According to some analysts these studies have been determined to be shoddy and full of major inaccuracies.[27] According to some analysts, the Bressler Report, compiled by the FDA in 1977, verifies the poor quality of the preapproval studies conducted on aspartame. An objective analysis of the data strongly supports the assertion that aspartame's approval by the FDA was based on manipulation, deception, and influential government leaders, and not scientific proof.

Just Who Owns Aspartame Anyway?

From 1965 to 1998, aspartame was a part of drugmaker G. D. Searle & Co. In 1998, Monsanto Company acquired G. D. Searle, and its aspartame business became a subsidiary company: the NutraSweet Company. Monsanto sold it to two companies: Merisant (a group of investors including Michael Dell of Dell Computers), which owns the brands Equal and Canderel®; and NutraSweet, which is owned by J. W. Childs Equity Partners, an investment firm in Boston[28] and its equity interests in two European joint venture companies to Ajinomoto Co. Inc.[29]

Annual sales of aspartame imploded after the patent expired, and manufacturers were abandoning it in droves because of the oversupply in the marketplace and the liability question.[30] Profits dropped from $1.5 billion per year to less than $150 million in 2003.

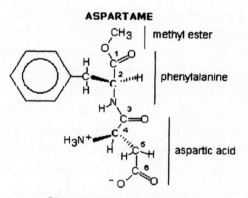

Diagram of Aspartame Molecule

Why Is Aspartame So Potentially Toxic?

Scientifically known as 1-aspartyl 1-phenylalanine methyl ester, aspartame has three components: phenylalanine, which makes up 50 percent of the chemical by weight; aspartic acid, which makes up 40 percent; and methanol (wood alcohol), which makes up 10 percent.[31] Those who defend this popular artificial sweetener state that the two primary amino acids, which make up 90 percent of aspartame, are a harmless and natural part of our diet. They insist that aspartic acid is a naturally occurring neurotransmitter that is present in the human central nervous system.

This, of course, is only a partial truth.

Phenylalanine and aspartic acid are amino acids that are normally supplied by the foods we eat; however, they can only be considered natural and harmless when they are consumed in combination with other amino acids (protein), fats, and carbohydrates in the form of genuine whole foods. When you eat foods in their natural state, protein, fats, and carbohydrates exist in an ideal relationship to each other and promote better health. When phenylalanine and aspartic acid are consumed as free-form amino acids, rather than with the full balance of amino acids found in foods, they enter your central nervous system in unusual and abnormally high concentrations, causing excessive firing of brain neurons and potential cell death. This concept has been termed *excitotoxicity* by Dr. Russell Blaylock, a prominent neurosurgeon in this field.

The neurotoxic effects of these amino acids, when consumed as free-form substances, are linked to headaches, mental confusion, balance problems, and seizures.[32-34] Additionally, what the manufacturers of aspartame are not telling us is that while aspartic acid and phenylalanine do naturally occur in food, they never occur isolated together and are attached as a single entity. The unique amino acid sequence of aspartic acid and phenylalanine does not occur anywhere in nature—and your body does not know what to do with it. Instead, your body recognizes it as a foreign chemical and attempts to metabolize and excrete it, which means aspartame and phenylalanine have the potential to wreak havoc in your body.[35]

ASPARTAME—THE WORLD'S BEST ANT POISON

"We live in the woods and carpenter ants are a huge problem. We have spent thousands of dollars with Orkin and on ant poisons trying to keep them under control but nothing has helped.

I opened two packets of aspartame sweetener, and dumped one in a corner of each of our bathrooms. That was about 2 years ago and I have not seen any carpenter ants for about 9 to 12 months. It works better than the most deadly poisons I have tried. Any time they show up again, I simply dump another package of Nutrasweet in a corner, and they will be gone for a year or so again.

Since posting this information I have had many people tell me of their success solving ant problems with this substance, when nothing else worked.

We found later that small black ants would not eat the aspartame. It was determined that if you mixed it with apple juice, they would quickly take it back to the nest, and all would be dead within 24 hours, usually.

How does it work: Aspartame is a neuropoison. It most likely kills the ants by interfering with their nervous system."[36]

Alarming Amino Acids and Aspartame

Amino acids are the name given to the basic structural unit of proteins. Nitrogen molecules are combined with hydrogen to make what is called an amino group. Each amino acid also has a carboxyl group, which is made up of carbon, oxygen, and hydrogen. Finally, amino acids have what is called an "R" group, which is a distinctive side group that makes each amino acid different from one another.

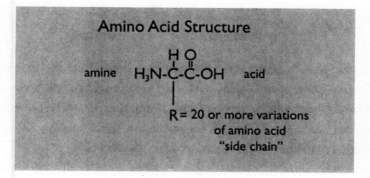

Diagram of Amino Acid

Amino groups and carboxyl groups are not chemically reactive. Essentially they are the stable part of an amino acid. The side chain is what characterizes an amino acid and ultimately determines its function. Amino acids can be charged or uncharged, acidic or basic. To date, more than three hundred different amino acids have been described in nature. Of the three hundred, only twenty are commonly found in mammals.

Recycled amino acids are called endogenous amino acids, or "nonessential" amino acids. They have been labeled as nonessential because your body has the ability to produce them through your own metabolic pathways, meaning they are not required as part of your diet. Essential amino acids are those that your body can't synthesize on its own. The only way to obtain essential amino acids is through what you eat. There are eight essential amino acids and twelve nonessentials.

Because amino acids are found naturally in food, your body is normally able to absorb them. However, in nature, amino acids do not exist alone but are found in combination with fats and carbohydrates. For example, a piece of meat may contain 4 percent phenylalanine in combination with a variety of other amino acids and fats.

As you will see, both phenylalanine and aspartic acid—the amino acid components of aspartame—have well-documented central nervous system toxicities. While it is certainly true that your body requires a small amount of these amino acids in order for your nervous system to function properly, when your body is given an overdose of these two amino acids taken in their free form and in combination with methanol, serious problems may ensue.

Yes, Aspartame Is Absorbed in Your Body

So what happens to aspartame after you have consumed it? The physical breakdown of protein and amino acids begins in your mouth as soon as you start chewing your food. Chewing signals your stomach to begin secreting enzymes and hydrochloric acid. This begins the direct process of breaking the peptide bonds that hold the amino acids together.

From here, smaller protein fractions enter your small intestine. Your pancreas releases a series of enzymes, such as cholecystokinin and secretin, which further break down the peptide bonds. Then, small peptides called oligopeptides, composed of between two and twelve amino acids, enter the cells that line your small intestine.

Free-form amino acids are absorbed by your intestinal cells and are broken down into other amino acids and various by-products before they enter your bloodstream. From here, the amino acids are either metabolized by your liver, or sent into your general circulation to be utilized by the rest of your body.

A large proportion of amino acids are absorbed and utilized immediately by the cells that line your small intestine. These intestinal cells are very metabolically active and feed upon specific amino acids.

Do You Really Want to Drink Wood Alcohol?

So yes, aspartame is fully absorbed into your bloodstream. Potentially most worrisome is the 10 percent of aspartame that is absorbed into your bloodstream as its breakdown product methanol (wood alcohol). The Environmental Protection Agency defines safe consumption of this dangerous substance as no more than 7.8 milligrams per day. And yet, a can of diet soda contains almost 16 milligrams of methanol.

But for most people, it's not the actual amino acids or methanol that causes the toxic side effects in your system, but the breakdown products they convert to on the shelf or as they are metabolized in your body. Phenylalanine decomposes into DKP, a known carcinogen, when it is exposed to warm temperatures or prolonged storage. And even if aspartame products are kept consistently at a cooler temperature, you're still at risk. Even at cold temperatures, methanol can spontaneously break down to a colorless toxin known as formaldehyde. Formaldehyde can accumulate within your cells and react with other cellular proteins such as enzymes and DNA. This cumulative reaction may result in severe consequences for those who consume diet drinks and aspartame-containing foods on a daily basis.[37]

The Dangers of Methanol Poisoning

Once swallowed, the methyl ester in aspartame is broken down into methanol (aka wood alcohol, paint remover), which is an extremely toxic substance. Your body further metabolizes methanol via an enzyme system in your liver called alcohol dehydrogenase. It is then broken down into formaldehyde, which your body has the potential to store before it is ultimately converted into the end waste product formate. In human and monkey studies, the accumulation of formate has been shown to be responsible for the production of metabolic acidosis (excessive acidity in the blood) in methanol poisoning. Methanol poisoning can result in fatal kidney damage, blindness, multiple organ system failure, and death.[38]

The manufacturers of aspartame defend the methanol produced in it by claiming it is found naturally in many foods. This partial truth is a clever deception, because methanol never exists bound to amino acids in nature. In fruit and fruit juices, for example, methanol is bound to pectin, which is a form of fiber. As a result of this bond, your body is not exposed to methanol, nor does it break it down. Your body excretes it before it is metabolized to formaldehyde.

The old saying, "An apple a day keeps the doctor away," like many adages, has some truth to it. Apples are loaded with pectin, which naturally helps your body clean itself by acting as a scouring abrasive in your digestive tract. When the pectin fiber progresses to your stool, it pulls items like methanol right along with it, so they are both eliminated from your body. In fact, according to Dr. James Bowen, MD, this quality of pectin is well known to many whose professions put them at risk of accidentally ingesting methanol, such as mechanics, and it works so well that when this happens they "will often successfully treat themselves by merely ingesting orange juice and going on about their work with no further problems."[39]

In addition, the natural methanol that is found in foods is always accompanied by ethanol (the alcohol found in beer and wine), which counteracts methanol's effects on the body. In fact, ethanol is the antidote to methanol poisoning. There is no ethanol in aspartame.[40, 41]

With aspartame, there is no natural binder for methanol once it is in your body. As a result, nearly all of the methanol is metabolically converted into formaldehyde, which is five thousand times more potent a poison than the ethyl alcohol you'd find in a glass of wine.[42] And what is worse is that methanol and phenylalanine both increase dopamine in the brain and can cause somewhat of a "high," which makes aspartame highly addictive.

Aspartame liberates free methyl alcohol, which causes chronic methanol poisoning. This, in turn, alters the dopamine levels in the brain and contributes to the addiction. Methanol is classified as a narcotic. People who have tried to quit aspartame have reported debilitating withdrawal symptoms including tension, irritability, tremors, nausea, depression, and sweating, which are ameliorated when aspartame consumption is resumed.[43-45]

Highly Hazardous Aspartame Breakdown Products Can Cause Cancer

Formaldehyde is the chemical used to preserve cadavers and is widely used in the industrial world to manufacture building materials and many household products. It is also a by-product of combustion and certain other natural processes. Formaldehyde, by itself or in combination with other chemicals, serves a number of purposes—for example, it is used to add permanent-press qualities to clothing and draperies, as a component of glues and adhesives, and as a preservative in some paints and coating products. It is also used in over a hundred different pesticides.

Sources of formaldehyde in the home or office include building materials, cigarettes, household products, and the use of unvented fuel-burning appliances like gas stoves or kerosene space heaters. Formaldehyde is normally present at low levels, usually less than 0.06 ppm (parts per million), in both outdoor and indoor air. When present in the air at levels at or above 0.1 ppm, acute health effects can occur including watery eyes, burning sensations in the eyes, nose, and throat, nausea, coughing, chest tightness, wheezing, skin rashes, and other irritating effects.

Formaldehyde affects people in various ways. Some people are very sensitive to formaldehyde, while others may have no noticeable reaction at the same level of exposure. Sensitive people can experience symptoms at levels below 0.1 ppm. The World Health Organization recommends that exposure should not exceed 0.05 ppm.[46]

According to the EPA, formaldehyde can cause cancer in laboratory animals and likely causes cancer in humans. There is no known threshold level below which there is no threat of cancer. The risk depends upon amount and duration of exposure.

In 1999, the *Western Journal of Medicine* had a report suggesting that since formaldehyde is a known inducer of cancer, because it alters DNA, anyone with breast and prostate cancer consuming aspartame should be concerned.[47]

The article showed a graph of breast cancer incidence against that of the rising consumption of aspartame. From the time that aspartame was first approved for limited use in 1974, expanded in 1981, and became unlimited in 1983, the breast cancer incidence went up dramatically along with the sharp peaks of increase in aspartame consumption over time. The same curve matched for rates of prostate cancer.

Aspartame—Hidden Cause of Headaches, Depression

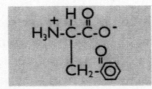

Diagram of Phenylalanine Molecule

Phenylalanine is one of two main amino acids in aspartame. In the "L" configuration, phenylalanine is converted naturally in the body to tyrosine, and subsequently L-dopa, norepinephrine, and epinephrine. These important neurotransmitters play a significant role in moderating brain chemistry. Excessive phenylalanine can alter the delicate balance of these neurotransmitter ratios and therefore cause a variety of neurological symptoms such as depression, anxiety attacks, tremors, headaches, and seizures. Because it affects brain chemistry, aspartame interacts with psychotropic medications including antidepressants.

Aspartame Causes Mental Retardation in Phenylketonuria (PKU)

Phenylalanine is commonly known in association with the genetic disease phenylketonuria (PKU), which occurs in one in five thousand births. PKU is characterized by the inability of the body to utilize phenylalanine, which causes a toxic buildup in the body that can lead to mental retardation unless proper care is taken. PKU is routinely screened for at birth.

People with PKU cannot, under any circumstance, eat any food containing phenylalanine, including aspartame. They are placed on a very strict diet that specifically excludes all aspartame products. The FDA has therefore required the manufacturers of aspartame to put warning labels on all of their products to protect consumers.

Aspartame, Aspartic Acid, and Brain Damage

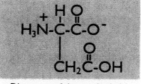

Diagram of Aspartic Acid

The other amino acid in aspartame is aspartic acid, which is a variant of the more commonly known amino acid aspartate. Aspartate is found naturally in plants, such as sprouting seeds, but is relatively uncommon in the human diet; it's a "nonessential" amino acid, so the body is able to make all the aspartate it needs.

In foods containing protein, aspartate exists mainly in the form of asparagine, not aspartic acid. Very rarely does anyone ever consume natural aspartate in its free form of aspartic acid.

In your body, aspartate (but not aspartic acid) plays an important role in the Kreb's cycle, which is responsible for producing energy for your brain, heart, and other important vital organs. So asparagine, the uncharged variant, is of therapeutic use in brain and neurological imbalances. This amino acid increases the resistance to fatigue, thereby stepping up the stamina of athletes. It also enhances the functioning of your liver.[48]

Aspartic acid, on the other hand, serves as a major excitatory neurotransmitter in your brain. Aspartic acid is frequently decreased in depressives and patients with brain atrophy, and it may be increased in people who experience seizures and strokes. In very high doses, aspartic acid also has the potential to cause brain damage.[49]

Excitotoxins Can Excite Your Cells to Death

As mentioned earlier, the concept of aspartame as an excitotoxin has led many to criticize its regular use in food products. Its potential for health complications in this arena is limitless.

Dr. John Olney, a neurophysiologist, showed that a single dose of mono-sodium glutamate (MSG), when given orally to rats or monkeys, raised blood glutamate levels to the point of causing brain damage in the hypothal-amus. This particular part of the brain is not well protected by the blood-brain barrier and appears to be more vulnerable to environmental toxins. While observing this, Dr. Olney coined the concept of excitotoxicity—the ability of amino acids such as glutamate and aspartic acid to literally excite nerve cells to death.[50]

Olney was able to convince food manufactures by bringing to their attention a study that was done on newborn animals. He found that new-borns were more susceptible to excitotoxic damage than adults were. In other studies he demonstrated that MSG caused certain nerve cells in the brain to die.[51]

Olney's early scientific efforts led him to ask the makers of baby food to remove MSG from all baby food products, which they did in an effort to protect consumers (and not be held liable). He then urged the FDA to ban MSG in children's food, but they did not comply. Unfortunately many foods that small children eat regularly, such as canned soup, still contain MSG.

Today, the concept of excitotoxins is universally accepted. The scientific community has even embraced the potential of excitotoxicity to lead to the development of neurodegenerative diseases such as Parkinson's and Alzheimer's. While this concept has become widely accepted, the FDA still refuses to recognize the danger of free-form amino acids acting as excito-toxins in foods. To date, they have not required any food manufacturers to remove potential excitotoxic amino acids from the food supply—MSG, aspartic acid, or any others.

Excitotoxins have also been shown to stimulate the generation of free radicals, which are charged molecules with an unpaired electron. Free radicals can seriously damage tissues and organs inside and outside your central nervous system. Evidence indicates that free radical production accelerates many degenerative illnesses such as atherosclerosis, cancer, coronary artery disease, and arthritis.[52, 53] It comes as no surprise that joint pain is a major complaint among those who have reported adverse reactions to aspartame.[54]

Your Blood-Brain Barrier—The Key to Protecting Your Brain

The blood-brain barrier (BBB) is a system of specialized capillary structures that are designed to prevent toxic substances from entering your brain. There are a number of medical conditions, including diabetes, hypertension, and simple aging, that may result in your blood-brain barrier becoming damaged and relatively "leaky." Smoking also can cause lasting damage to this delicate barrier. Aspartame reactions may have a tendency to be magnified in individuals with these types of health conditions.

In utero, and during the first twelve months of life, your blood-brain barrier is incomplete and not well insulated. As a result, excitotoxins, including aspartic acid, have free access to enter your central nervous system. Experimentally, it has been determined that infants are four times more sensitive to excitotoxins than adults.[55] It has been scientifically proven that during the first year of life, irreversible brain damage can occur through chemical agents that have contaminated breast milk and crossed the BBB. In spite of this, the American Dietetic Association, the Calorie Control Council, and the American Diabetes Association all approve the use aspartame and other artificial sweeteners for pregnant and lactating women.[56] Not surprisingly, however, as you'll find out in chapter 5, several of those organizations are nothing more than front groups for corporate interests.

The Federation of American Societies for Experimental Biology (FASEB), which usually mimics the FDA's opinions, recently stated in a review:

> It is prudent to avoid the use of dietary supplements of L-glutamic acid by pregnant women, infants, and children. The existence of evidence of potential endocrine responses, i.e., elevated cortisol and prolactin, and differential responses between males and females, would also suggest a neuroendocrine link and that supplemental L-glutamic acid should be avoided by women of childbearing age and individuals with affective disorders.[57]

The aspartic acid in aspartame has been shown to have the same deleterious effects on the body as glutamic acid.

The concentrating effects of the placenta are also able to magnify the levels of phenylalanine in the blood by as much as four- to sixfold in a fetus.[58]

Fetal phenylalanine has the potential to reach levels that kill cells in tissue culture. It's not much of a stretch to theorize that these concentrations harbor the threat of birth defects in the developing infant. There are enormous risks to infants, children, pregnant women, the elderly, and people with certain chronic health problems.

Research Studies: The Good, the Bad, and the Ugly

A number of books and extensive review articles have been published on the research that has been conducted on aspartame. For a complete list of all studies ever published on aspartame, the National Library Medline Index can be used. As of July 2006, there were 816 published studies on aspartame indexed in the National Library of Medicine.[59]

Because aspartame has been implicated in so many different disease states, the information that follows will be limited to studies that have found aspartame to be a definite causative factor.

Aspartame and Migraines

Despite the FDA approval for aspartame as an all-purpose sweetener, many doctors and researchers in the scientific community remain skeptical. They expressly remain cautious regarding individuals who suffer from migraines, epilepsy, and neuropsychiatric problems. In recent years there have been several studies demonstrating an exacerbation in headaches with aspartame consumption.

Three randomized double-blind, placebo-controlled studies—the gold standard of medicine—have been conducted involving more than two hundred adult migraine sufferers and lasting between fourteen and twenty-four days.[60-62] Headaches were more frequent and more severe in the aspartame-treated group when compared to controls. In a fourth study that failed to confirm that aspartame caused migraines, aspartame consumption only occurred for one day, hardly the amount of time typically required to demonstrate toxicity exposures.[63]

The evidence appears to be quite clear that aspartame use triggers headaches in individuals who suffer from migraines, particularly when there is prolonged consumption. The outcome here is nondebatable: if you have headaches, avoid aspartame.

Aspartame and Cancer

One of the most serious accusations against aspartame is its possible link to brain cancer. While this subject remains a controversial one, there are some facts that we can reference. Dr. John Olney, the neurologist cited earlier in the section on excitotoxins, published an article in the *Journal of Neuropathology and Experimental Neurology*, looking at rates of brain cancer in relation to the inauguration of aspartame.[64] Following FDA approval in 1983, over six million pounds of aspartame were consumed in the form of diet soda. In January of 1984, brain cancer rates began to skyrocket at an alarmingly faster rate than any other form of cancer. This was happening at the same time that many other types of cancers were beginning to decrease in incidence.

Olney hypothesized that the increasing rates of brain cancer could be due to the introduction of aspartame. This hypothesis was supported by an FDA trial in 320 rats, in which twelve rats developed malignant brain tumors after receiving aspartame-containing feed for two years.[65]

The response of the aspartame's manufacturers was swift. Several individuals wrote editorials in an attempt to dismiss Olney's hypothesis. They claimed that several other factors could also be influencing the increased rates of brain cancer, including depletion of the ozone layer and the use of home computers, cordless telephones, and VCRs. However, none of those theories explains the immediate increase following aspartame's introduction into the food chain.

According to the National Cancer Institute, there was a 10 percent increase in the incidence of common primary malignant brain cancer in 1985, and perhaps as early as 1984. This phenomenon occurred one to two years following the approval of aspartame for beverages in July 1983. It includes a disproportionately high rise in alioblastoma, astrocytoma, and primary lymphoma among young women who consume large amounts of aspartame-containing beverages. There has also been an increased occurrence of cancer in the brain and spinal cord among children whose mothers consumed aspartame throughout their pregnancy.[66, 67]

More recently, Dr. Morando Soffritti, a cancer researcher in Bologna, Italy, who has spent twenty-eight years doing research on potential carcinogens, performed a study that found aspartame was associated with an unusually high rate of lymphomas, leukemias, and other cancers in rats that had been given doses of it starting at what would be equivalent to four to five twenty-ounce bottles of diet soda a day for a 150-pound person. The study was published in a medical journal financed by the National Institute of Health.[68]

Dr. Soffritti was inspired to look at aspartame because of inadequacies in the cancer studies done by Searle in the 1970s. He was concerned about the large numbers of people who use aspartame, particularly children and pregnant women. Unfortunately, as of the date this book was written, no regulatory agency has yet acted on Dr. Soffritti's findings.

The Delaney Clause states that "[n]o additive shall be deemed to be safe if it is found to induce cancer when ingested by man or animal, or if it is found, after tests which are appropriate for the evaluation of the safety of food additives, to induce cancer in man or animal." In other words, if a food additive causes cancer, it is illegal to add it to food.[69] In 1985, the late FDA toxicologist Dr. Adrian Gross testified to the Senate:

> In view of all these indications that the cancer-causing potential of aspartame is a matter that had been established way beyond any reasonable doubt, one can ask: What is the reason for the apparent refusal by the FDA to invoke for this food additive the so-called Delaney Amendment to the Food, Drug and Cosmetic Act? Is it not clear beyond any shadow of a doubt that aspartame has caused brain tumors or brain cancer in animals?[70]

We are still waiting for an answer as our cancer rates continue to climb each year.

Aspartame Can Cause Depression and Other Brain Injuries

Because aspartame is known to affect the nervous system, it should come as no surprise that it has been implicated as a causative factor for depression in certain populations.[71] It has been reported that as much as two-thirds of aspartame reactions involve neurologic or behavioral symptoms—although the reports are generally anecdotal, and often double-blind studies fail to replicate these reactions.

However, it has been demonstrated that aspartame can significantly increase rat brain phenylalanine levels, and that it can, in combination with carbohydrates, raise brain tyrosine levels. This ultimately suppresses the usual increase in brain tryptophan levels that would ordinarily follow a carbohydrate-rich meal. Changes in neurotransmitters can have a significant impact on your nervous system and may ultimately lead to depression in some individuals.

Dr. Walton, of Northeastern Ohio University, decided to examine the connection with a double-blind study.[72] The original trial was to study forty patients with depression and forty control patients with no history of depression. But the project was halted by the Institutional Review Board after a total of thirteen individuals from the depressive group dropped out of the study because of the severity of their reactions.

One person who left the study suffered from a detached retina that ultimately led to permanent blindness. He had used aspartame for the first time during the course of the study. Another patient suffered from a bleeding conjunctiva in her eye. (In a 1988 study, it was reported that of 505 aspartame reactors, 35 percent complained of eye pain or visual changes.[73]) Three patients reported feeling as if "they were poisoned."

It's reasonable to conclude that individuals with mood disorders are particularly sensitive to this artificial sweetener and should avoid it.

As an interesting aside, Dr. Walton notes that in the planning phases of his trial, the NutraSweet Company refused to sell him aspartame for use in the study.[74]

They told him that the raw material was not available for him to experiment with; he had to go to a supplier other than the manufacturing company to obtain the raw material. There are many implications from the NutraSweet Company's refusal to sell aspartame to a researcher.

Aspartame and Epilepsy/Seizures

Seizure development appears to be one of the primary side effects caused by aspartame consumption. Most individuals affected this way have no prior history of seizures and have no further seizures after stopping aspartame. At the Massachusetts Institute of Technology, eighty people who had suffered seizures after ingesting aspartame were surveyed. Community Nutrition Institute concluded the following about the survey:

> These 80 cases meet the FDA's own definition of an imminent hazard to the public health, which requires the FDA to expeditiously remove a product from the market.[75]

Even the U.S. Military Warns Its Pilots Against Using Aspartame

Both the air force's magazine *Flying Safety* and the navy's magazine *Navy Physiology* published articles warning about the many dangers of aspartame use.[76] The articles note that the ingestion of aspartame can make pilots more susceptible to seizures and vertigo.

The United States Air Force went on to warn all pilots to stay off aspartame, stating:

> Some people have suffered aspartame related disorders with doses as small as that carried in a single stick of chewing gum. This could mean a pilot who drinks diet sodas is more susceptible to flicker vertigo, or flicker-induced epileptic activity. It also means that all pilots are potential victims of sudden memory loss, dizziness during instrument flight and gradual loss of vision.[77]

Twenty articles sounding warnings about ingesting aspartame while flying have also appeared in the *National Business Aircraft Association Digest* (1993), *Aviation Medical Bulletin* (1988), *The Aviation Consumer* (1988), *Canadian General Aviation News* (1990), *Pacific Flyer* (1988), *General Aviation News* (1989), *Aviation Safety Digest* (1989), and *Plane and Pilot* (1990), and a paper warning about aspartame was presented at the 57th Annual Meeting of the Aerospace Medical Association (Gaffney 1986).

Shortly after these articles became publicly available, a hotline was set up for pilots suffering from acute reactions to aspartame ingestion. Over six hundred pilots have reported symptoms, including some who have reported suffering grand mal seizures in the cockpit due to aspartame.

Aspartame and Vision Impairment

You'll recall the bizarre story of upside-down Peter at the beginning of the chapter. The individual components of aspartame, as well as their multiple breakdown products, are potentially toxic to your retina and optic nerves. Methanol poisoning has a reputation for causing vision impairment, which may lead to blindness.[78] The classic pattern of methanol toxicity includes an initial central nervous system depression, followed by a latent period of ten to thirty hours. After this asymptomatic period, a syndrome usually develops that is characterized primarily by visual impairment. This impairment may range from blurring to complete vision loss.

Formaldehyde, the primary metabolite of methanol, is also known to cause retinal damage. Aspartame has been linked to visual disturbances including blindness in one or both eyes, blurred visibility, eye pain, and more. Visual hallucinations have also been noted in many individuals.

Dr. H. J. Roberts, MD, has written extensively about aspartame and treated hundreds of aspartame reactors. A quarter of his patients have experienced decreased vision or blindness. According to Dr. Roberts, the optic nerve swelling, retinal degeneration, and visual impairment associated with heavy aspartame use is identical to the pathology observed in recorded cases of methanol toxicity from drinking wood alcohol throughout the days of prohibition.[79]

Can Aspartame Cause You to Gain Weight?

Research has shown aspartame may cause weight *gain*. One reason for this is phenylalanine and aspartic acid, amino acids which make up the bulk of aspartame, are known to rapidly stimulate the release of insulin and leptin, which are hormones that signal the body to store fat. Additionally, large doses of phenylalanine can lower important neurotransmitters like serotonin, which signals your body to tell it that it is satiated. Low levels of serotonin can then lead to food cravings, which can result in an increase in carbohydrate cravings that ultimately lead to weight gain.[80]

In a study of high-intensity use of artificial sweeteners performed on college students, there was no evidence that artificial sweetener use was associated with a decrease in their sugar intake. These results indicate that eating artificial sweeteners simply perpetuates a craving for sweets, and overall sugar consumption is not reduced—leading to further problems controlling your weight.[81]

Another study based on eight years of epidemiological data showed that drinking soft drinks increased the likelihood of weight gain by 65 percent, but it was the *diet* soda that was associated with "serious weight gain," not the regular soda. This finding was replicated in a study at Purdue University, which found that rats fed diet soda ate more high-calorie food than rats that were fed a drink sweetened with a high-caloric sweetener. According to nutritional expert Leslie Beck, "Your taste buds may be temporarily satisfied by the sweet taste of a diet pop, but your brain isn't fooled, and it still wants to make up for calories later on."[82]

Aspartame and Neurological Diseases

Aspartame has been shown to cause holes in the brains of rats. This is why neurological symptoms are so common in aspartame users. Dr. H. J. Roberts, the foremost medical authority on aspartame, said that he has had many patients in their thirties and forties consult with him for symptoms of Alzheimer's. They were confused, forgetful, couldn't think. Once they stopped using aspartame, their symptoms disappeared. Dr. Roberts believes that aspartame is partially responsible for the widespread epidemic of Alzheimer's in the United States, because it speeds up the process.[83]

According to Dr. Russell Blaylock, author of *Excitotoxins: The Taste That Kills*, excitotoxins may be a contributing factor in the development of Parkinson's disease. Excitotoxins, like aspartic acid (in aspartame) and glutamate (in MSG), excessively stimulate the brain cells, which then generate free radicals causing cell injury and even death. The reason why everyone does not develop neurological disorders from excitotoxins is because some individuals (e.g. those who eat a diet low in nutrients and antioxidants) have cellular defense enzymes that are either immature or defective, and are unable to protect the brain cells from the excitotoxins.[84]

The additional toxins in aspartame—DKP, aspartate, methanol, formaldehyde, and formic acid—also act as neurotoxins in the brain. Recent evidence demonstrates that the aspartame product formaldehyde accumulates within cells and damages protein and DNA.[85]

Side effects from formaldehyde exposure include:

- Irreversible genetic damage from long-term, low-level exposure (Shaham 1996)

- Headaches, fatigue, chest tightness (Main 1983)

- Sleeping problems, burning skin, fatigue, chest pain, dizziness (Liu 1991)

- Headaches, fatigue, IgE-mediated sensitization (Wantke 1996)

- Musculoskeletal, gastrointestinal, and cardiovascular symptoms (Srivastava 1992)

- Headaches, tiredness (Olsen 1982)

- Headaches, dizziness, nausea, lack of concentration ability (Burdach 1980)

- Cytogenic effects of blood lymphocytes (Suruda 1993)

- Fertility (adverse effects) (Taskinen 1999)

- Cognitive adverse effects (Kilburn 2000)

- Seizures and neurobehavioral impairment (Kilburn 1994)

- Headaches, skin problems (Proietti 2002)

- Low birth weight (Maroziene 2002)

- Neurobehavioral symptoms (Kilburn 1985)

- Memory problems, equilibrium and dexterity impairment (Kilburn 1987)[86]

The Cost of Aspartame on the Environment

According to Scorecard.org, a pollution information site, the NutraSweet Company's aspartame manufacturing facility in Augusta, Georgia, ranks in the 80–90 percentile among U.S. factories for the worst polluter for total environmental releases and cancer risk score. They also ranked in the 90–100 percentile for air releases of recognized developmental toxicants (toxicants that cause adverse effects on the developing child).[87]

2002 RANKINGS: MAJOR CHEMICAL RELEASES OR WASTE GENERATION AT THIS FACILITY

Cleanest/Best Facilities in US					Percentile		Dirtiest/Worst Facilities in US			
0%	10%	20%	30%	40%	50%	60%	70%	80%	90%	100%

Total environmental releases

Cancer risk score (air and water releases):

Noncancer risk score (air and water releases):

Air releases of recognized developmental toxicants:

Scorce: Scorecard.org

Also in 2002, the NutraSweet Company shipped off nearly *twenty-million pounds of hazardous waste* to the landfill—including chlorodifluoromethane, a known ozone depleter, and chloromethane, a chemical known to be a major contributor to cancer risk. These contaminants are being released into the environment daily.[88]

Not only is consuming NutraSweet very likely harmful to you personally, but making it (and purchasing it) comes at an enormous cost to the environment.

Other artificial sweeteners are similarly dangerous for the environment. As you will see in the next chapter, the Tate & Lyle Splenda factory in McIntosh, Alabama, is equally devastating to the ecosystem and the people who live in the community.

Next in Line

Is neotame just another form of aspartame? Unfortunately, the answer is yes. Neotame is a modified version that contains the same two amino acids, aspartic acid and L-phenylalanine, as well as two other organic compounds, a methyl ester and a neohexyl group. The close similarity means that most of the dangers of aspartame you've just read about are likely to pertain to neotame as well.

Neotame is currently found primarily in chewing gum, carbonated sodas, candy, yogurts, baked goods, and frozen desserts. Its use is likely to spread over the next few years.

At Least One Million May Have Had
Side Effects from Aspartame

For anyone who doubts the frequency of aspartame reactions, the FDA has received over ten thousand complaints submitted by people who have had them. In February 1994, the U.S. Department of Health and Human Services released an extensive list (see Appendix B) of aspartame-induced reactions, which encompassed everything from chronic fatigue syndrome and seizures to infertility and death.

In 1988, 80 percent of the calls that were made to the FDA to complain about foods and food additives were about aspartame-related adverse reactions. In 2002 alone, the European Scientific Committee on Food received over five hundred complaints concerning aspartame reactions.[89]

By the FDA's own admission, less than 1 percent of those who experience a reaction to a product ever report it. This means that the ten thousand documented accounts probably indicate that there are roughly a million people who have experienced reactions to aspartame.[90] Most victims are not aware that aspartame may be at the root of their problems, and end up spending a tremendous amount of time and money trying to figure out why they are sick.

While a variety of symptoms have been reported, almost two-thirds of them fall into the neurological/behavioral category consisting mostly of headache, mood alteration, and hallucination. The remaining third is comprised mostly of gastrointestinal symptoms. The following list will provide you with the most common reported symptoms associated with aspartame consumption (for a complete list, see appendix B):

Side Effects of Aspartame[91]

Headache	Dizziness/poor equilibrium
Change in mood	Hallucination
Vomiting or nausea	Abdominal pain and cramps
Change in vision	Diarrhea
Seizures and convulsions	Memory loss
Fatigue, weakness	Rash
Sleep problems/insomnia	Hives
Change in heart rate	

How to Determine if You React to Aspartame

One of the best ways to determine if you are having a reaction to aspartame, or any other artificial sweetener, is to perform an elimination/challenge with it. First, eliminate it and all other artificial sweeteners from your diet completely for a period of one to two weeks. After this period, reintroduce it in a significant quantity.

For example, use it in your beverage in the morning and eat at least two aspartame-containing products the remainder of the day. Avoid other artificial sweeteners on this day so that you are able to differentiate which one may be causing a problem for you. Do this for a period of one to three days. Notice how your body is feeling, particularly if it feels different than when you were artificial-sweetener free. Nearly two-thirds of aspartame reactors experienced symptomatic improvement within two days after avoiding aspartame. With continued abstinence, their complaints generally disappeared.

Please note that if you are discontinuing diet sodas with caffeine you will have to carefully reduce your use, as it is very common to suffer caffeine withdrawal. If this is a problem for you, please eliminate the diet soda more gradually.

If you complete the elimination/challenge trial described above and do not notice any changes, then it would appear you are able to tolerate artificial sweeteners acutely. However, please understand that this does not mean you are completely out of the woods and not being damaged by this artificial sweetener. The impact that artificial sweeteners will have on your long-term health has not yet been determined, especially when sweeteners are used in combination with each other.

Aspartame and Sucralose (Splenda)

The primary difference between aspartame and sucralose is that the base of aspartame is a combination of two amino acids, while the base of sucralose is derived from sugar, which is a carbohydrate.

There are, however, many similarities between the two:

- They are both manufactured chemicals with questionable roads to FDA approval.

- The majority of the research conducted on both aspartame and sucralose was performed by the companies that manufacture them, which clearly demonstrates a powerful conflict of interest.

- Many of the published studies make hypothetical assumptions based on the outcomes. Essentially, it's assumed that human studies would yield the same results as the animal studies. In addition, when a study outcome presents potential health concerns, the findings are explained away, rationalized, or dismissed as being of no consequence.

- No specific health benefits that result from consuming these products, as opposed to the health benefits gained from consuming nutrient rich, natural, whole foods.

- Both of these sweeteners were found accidentally in laboratories looking to make chemicals, not food.

And finally, as you'll see in the next chapter, Splenda, like aspartame, may be hazardous to your health.

CHAPTER FOUR: SWEET IGNORANCE

THE UNEXAMINED DANGERS OF SPLENDA

BETH'S STORY

Last January, Beth began to experience episodes during which she spontaneously fell down, seemingly for no reason at all. She would often wake up with her heart racing. She also battled many gastrointestinal symptoms such as extreme nausea, acid reflux, and alternating diarrhea and constipation. Numbness would occur in different areas of her body, and she also developed a three-inch circular rash on one side of her face.

Beth was terrified of these symptoms, so she went to numerous doctors and underwent many diagnostic tests. Her doctors could not determine the cause but suggested it was anxiety related. One day Beth realized that just before her symptoms began, she had switched to a "low carb diet" and had begun eating and drinking various sugar-free items and low-carb foods, many of which contained Splenda (sucralose). She discovered that whenever she drank or ate something with sucralose in it, she'd have panic attacks with simultaneous numbness and tingling in different areas of her body, typically within a few hours, but sometimes a day or two later. She decided to stop eating food with Splenda for a short time to see if it made a difference. Slowly but surely, her symptoms subsided and then almost completely disappeared.

Beth decided to retry one of her favorite sugar-free treats, just to be sure. A couple of days later, she had another attack almost identical to the ones she had experienced before. Since then, she has decided to stay away from anything sweetened with Splenda or sucralose for good.

Splenda

Splenda is the trade name of an artificial sweetener that has pulled off one of the most successful consumer product launches in history. It is currently the nation's number one selling artificial sweetener.[1]

Between 2000 and 2004, the percentage of U.S. households using Splenda products jumped from 3 percent to 20 percent.[2] Its sales have grown 126 percent over the past two years, and in 2005 retail sales of Splenda topped $187 million. On the other hand, rival sugar substitutes have declined by 8 percent, and 2005 retail sales were only $57 million for aspartame-based Equal and $51 million for saccharin-based Sweet'N Low.[3]

Splenda sales would be even higher, but the demand has actually outstripped the current supply. The manufacturer of Splenda is making additions to its current factory and is in the process of building new ones.

Splenda is found in over 4,500 products available in supermarkets and restaurants, from Starbucks to Jamba Juice. It is the primary sweetener in the new low-carb food and drinks made popular by the Atkins® and South Beach® diets.

LIST OF APPROVED USES FOR SPLENDA (SUCRALOSE)[4]

Baked goods and baking mixes	Beverages and beverage bases
Chewing gum	Coffee and tea
Sugar substitutes (for table use)	Fats and oils (salad dressing)
Frozen dairy desserts (ice cream)	Fruit and water ices
Gelatins, puddings, and fillings	Jams and jellies
Milk products	Processed fruits and fruit juices

Splenda is in products that you are drinking and that your children are eating. Not only is it found in food, but it is also hidden in chewing gum, pharmaceuticals, and a shockingly large number of "natural" health products, as many in the health food industry have fallen prey to Splenda's deceptive marketing campaign. This perceived endorsement by many in natural health industry tends to further reinforce the use of this chemical sweetener.

Part of the reason for Splenda's success is that it doesn't have the bitter metallic aftertaste of other artificial sweeteners, so it's disguised more easily in everything from candy bars to kettle corn. Another important reason for Splenda's rising popularity is that many manufacturers are abandoning the use of aspartame because of the health concerns and controversy surrounding it, such as the proposed ban of aspartame by the state of New Mexico.[5] Some aspartame distributors, such as Holland Sweeteners, have withdrawn from the U.S. market due to too many distributors and not enough demand.[6]

Just as aspartame inserted itself into the gap in the market created by the controversy over saccharin, Splenda has neatly positioned itself to take advantage of the growing body of evidence regarding the dangers of aspartame.

What Is Splenda?

Splenda is the brand name for sucralose, a chlorinated artificial sugar derivative up to six hundred times sweeter than sugar, with no calories and no carbohydrates. You can find sucralose in many manufactured products, but you as a consumer cannot buy sucralose by itself, as it is only available to manufacturers in quantities of no less than one kilogram at a cost of over $450/kilogram. Splenda products, which are the versions available to consumers, consist of sucralose combined with other caloric sweeteners, so that they measure and pour just like sugar.

SPLENDA PRODUCTS FOR CONSUMERS

> **Splenda No Calorie Sweetener:** Available in granular form and packets, this is a blend of sucralose with the sugars maltodextrin and/or dextrose.

Splenda Sugar Blend for Baking: This is a blend of sucralose and table sugar. It has the same number of calories per pound as table sugar, but you only need to use half as much because of its intense sweetness. Its texture in the finished products or recipes is inferior to sugar, as is its taste.

Splenda Brown Sugar Blend: This is similar to previous sugar blend except that it contains brown sugar instead of table sugar.

Sucralose—A Serendipitous Surprise

Sucralose, as we briefly mentioned in chapter 2, was discovered by accident, just like aspartame and so many other artificial sweeteners. In 1975, Shashikant Phadnis, an Indian graduate student in the chemistry department of Queen Elizabeth College in London, was working with his advisor, Leslie Hough, in their chemistry lab. They were trying to create new *insecticides*. The experiment involved taking sulfuryl chloride—a highly poisonous chemical—and adding it drop by drop to a sugar solution. This volatile reaction gave birth to 1′,4,6,6′-tetrachloro-1′,4,6,6′-tetradeoxygalactosucrose. These powders had molecules full of chlorine atoms. DDT, a proven *toxin*, also has many chlorine atoms.

At one point in the procedure, Hough asked Phadnis to *test* the powder, but Phadnis thought Hough was telling him to *taste* it. He told Hough that it was sweet.

"When I reported my findings to Les, he asked if I was *crazy* . . . how could I taste compounds without knowing anything about their toxicity?" However, not long after, Hough was so excited about their serendipitous discovery, he added some to his coffee.

It was Phadnis this time who warned Hough about the unknown toxicity. "Oh, forget it," Hough replied, "We'll survive!"[7]

Hough and Phadnis teamed up with a British sugar company, Tate & Lyle, to experiment on hundreds of chlorinated sugars before they finally selected one. Substituting three chlorine ions for three hydroxyl groups on a sugar molecule resulted in the artificial chemical whose name is "1,6-dichloro-1,6-dideoxy-beta-D-fructofuranosyl-4-chloro-4-deoxy-alpha-D-galactopyranoside".[8] We can only assume this molecule was then renamed "sucralose" to make it sound more natural.

In 1980, four years after the discovery of sucralose, Tate & Lyle sold the manufacturing rights of sucralose to Johnson & Johnson, one of the world's largest healthcare and pharmaceutical companies. Johnson & Johnson created a new company (McNeil Nutritionals LLC) to be solely responsible for Splenda marketing and production. In 2004, McNeil Nutritionals and Tate & Lyle restructured their alliance so that McNeil is now responsible for the marketing of Splenda brand products while Tate & Lyle is responsible for manufacturing sucralose.[9]

How Sucralose Was Introduced into the United States

In 1991, Canada became the first country to approve the use of sucralose. In the United States, on the other hand, sucralose was denied approval by the FDA for eleven years (1987–1998).[10]

Insiders say the approval of sucralose was delayed for over a decade because other artificial sweetener companies didn't want the competition and prevented it from being approved. Senator Harlan Mathews complained about the delay, arguing that "any third party could indefinitely delay approval of [a food] additive simply by repeatedly submitting their interpretation of data."[11]

An article in *Food Chemistry News* stated:

> The tardy submission . . . of old data about sucralose, data which purportedly was received from an anonymous source, may have reflected bad faith intervention by a company seeking to retain its competitive advantage in the market for non-nutritive sweeteners.[12]

According to two food industry insiders we interviewed, it was no coincidence that sucralose was suddenly approved around the same time Monsanto was asking for FDA approval of aspartame's chemical cousin, neotame. The competition stopped protesting the approval of sucralose for fear that McNeil would try to sabotage the approval of neotame.[13] In any case, with no warning, the FDA suddenly approved sucralose on April 1, 1998 (April Fools Day—how appropriate). After evaluating all the data in McNeil's petition and other information, the FDA concluded that the proposed uses of sucralose were safe. McNeil was caught off-guard by the sudden approval and had to scramble to build a facility that could meet the demand.[14]

Neotame was approved as a general use sweetener in 2002 without protest. It was a win-win scenario for everyone involved.

Everyone, that is, but the general public.

Diet R. C. Cola, introduced in May 1998, was the first U.S. product containing sucralose. The initial approval was for the use of sucralose in fifteen food and beverage categories, which is the broadest initial approval ever granted by the FDA for any food additive.[15] The FDA required no warnings or informational labels on products containing sucralose, although such warnings have been found on most other artificial sweeteners.

On August 12, 1999, a mere sixteen months after the initial approval of sucralose, the FDA approved sucralose for use as a general-purpose sweetener. Instead of moving forward cautiously and conducting independent human studies, sucralose was given unlimited access for inclusion in nearly every kind of food and beverage. Currently, sucralose has been approved for use in forty countries, including Canada, Australia, and Mexico, as well as the United States.

The FDA's final ruling noted that no adverse health effects were attributed to sucralose given to animals at doses hundreds of times higher than the maximum estimated intakes in humans. However, most taste research scientists interviewed for a recent article on sucralose refuse to eat it.

One of them commented, "I look at that structure and I have an irrational fear of it. I've seen the safety studies, and you feed it to rats and mice forever and nothing happens. But it just *scares me.*"

—Burkhard Bilger, reporter for the *New Yorker* magazine[16]

"Made From Sugar, So It Tastes Like Sugar"

McNeil Nutritionals has gone to great lengths to suggest that Splenda is natural and safe by using the slogan, "Made from sugar, so it tastes like sugar." But after the sugar has been treated with trityl chloride, acetic anhydride, hydrogen chlorine, thionyl chloride,. and methanol, in the presence of dimethylformamide, 4-methylmorpholine, toluene, methyl isobutyl ketone, acetic acid, benzyltriethlyammonium chloride, and sodium methoxide, it is anything but a sugar molecule.

THE FIVE-STEP PROCESS FOR CREATING
SUCRALOSE (SPLENDA)[17]

Splenda International Patent A23L001:

1. Sucrose is tritylated with trityl chloride in the presence of dimethylformamide and 4-methylmorpholine, and the tritylated sucrose is then acetylated with acetic anhydride.

2. The resulting sucrose molecule TRISPA (6,1',6'-tri-O-trityl-penta-O acetylsucrose) is chlorinated with hydrogen chlorine in the presence of toluene.

3. The resulting 4-PAS (sucrose 2,3,4,3',4'-pentaacetate) is heated in the presence of methyl isobutyl ketone and acetic acid.

4. The resulting 6-PAS (sucrose 2,3,6,3',4'-pentaacetate) is chlorinated with thionyl chloride in the presence of toluene and benzyltriethlyammonium chloride.

5. The resulting TOSPA (sucralose pentaacetate) is treated with methanol in the presence of sodium methoxide to produce sucralose.

Nowhere in nature is there any form of sugar that remotely resembles the resulting chlorinated hydrocarbon known as sucralose. This product is not natural, nor is it a real sugar. It isn't even close.

The patented process may seem to be a bit technical. It is. That's because sucralose is a chemical and not a food; it was discovered in the course of research on *insecticides,* not foodstuffs.

Sucrose, or table sugar, as you'll remember from chapter 1, is a disaccharide, composed of glucose and fructose, two simple sugars (monosaccharides). In the manufacturing process, along with the addition of chlorine, sucralose is transformed from a sucrose (fructo-*glucose*) molecule into a fructo-*galactose* molecule. The chemical structure of the original sugar molecule is so seriously manipulated that it changes to a different type of molecule altogether.

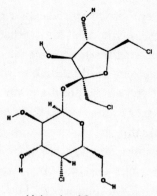

Molecule of Sucralose

It's important to understand that in nature, all disaccharides contain two sugar units, one of which is always a glucose unit. Since sucralose has no glucose unit, it's a brand-new creature, never before seen in nature. This is one of the reasons that your body doesn't have the enzymes to digest it. There has never been a need for your body to develop the metabolic machinery to digest this type of artificial molecule, because it has never existed before.

This is how McNeil Nutritionals justifies calling Splenda a nonnutritive, noncaloric sweetener. McNeil contends that it "just passes right through your body." As you will read later on, however, the digestive process of sucralose is much more complicated than that.

It's Clearly Unnatural—But Is It Also Unsafe?

You may have seen the full-page four-color Splenda ads proclaiming, "Think sugar, say Splenda," that have been placed in a wide variety of print media, including professional medical journals. These ads are aimed at assuring physicians of Splenda's safety, and encourage them to recommend it to their patients as a healthy alternative to sugar.

When I come across these ads, I'm strongly reminded of the cigarette advertisements placed in medical journals in the early 1900s, which encouraged physicians to *recommend* smoking to their patients. I suspect, just as with smoking today, one hundred years from now your descendants will be equally appalled when they hear that Splenda was once promoted to physicians for patient use. In the meantime, why should you needlessly put your health at risk?

Some of you have never touched Splenda and never will but are reading this to stay informed. Some of you don't know what to think and are looking to this book to tell you whether or not Splenda is safe. Some of you are looking for flaws in my arguments and research so you can continue to enjoy using it without worry. If you are skeptical and do not want to believe the case against Splenda, let me caution you to be as objective as possible and use common sense in evaluating this information.

Ask yourself this question: do you really believe you were designed to eat any artificial sweetener hundreds to thousands of times sweeter than sugar and not have any health consequences? I ask you to open your mind to the possibility that the manufacturers of these chemical compounds may NOT have your best health interests at the top of their priority list. Take all of this into account so you can make the best decision for your own health and the health of your family.

LUCY'S STORY

Lucy had experienced damaging side effects while using aspartame. So she was excited when she learned about Splenda; she thought that since it was "made from sugar," it wouldn't have the usual side effects associated with artificial sweeteners.

Lucy's main source of Splenda was in her daily low-carb desserts such as ice cream and cookies. She started to experience frequent headaches soon after she ate her dessert. They weren't as debilitating as the aspartame headaches, but they certainly set her back.

However, Lucy also began to experience episodes of anxiety and deep depression and began to have frequent thoughts of committing suicide. She noticed that her headaches and depression were much worse in the evening after she had her nightly Splenda dessert following dinner.

Lucy began to pay closer and closer attention to her symptoms and determined that they *only occurred after an exposure to Splenda.* She stopped using Splenda and other sucralose-containing products, and her headaches, anxiety, and depression have completely disappeared.

What You Need to Know About Chlorine

Chlorine (Cl) is a chemical element, a member of the halogen family of the periodic table. Free chlorine is not found in nature. It is artificially produced in factories by running an electric current in salt water. The result is a heavy, yellow, irritating gas that is highly toxic to life even at very low concentrations. According to the EPA, chlorine is a class-one carcinogen (cancer-causing agent) in humans.[18]

Chlorine has a long list of industrial uses. It is used alone as a bleaching agent and disinfectant or in combination with other chemicals to make anything from pesticides to plastics. It was used as a poisonous gas in World War I. An estimated 92,000 soldiers died, and another 1.2 million were hospitalized as a result of poison gas attacks.[19]

Chlorine has a notorious reputation because of all the harm it has caused to human health and the environment. Greenpeace has launched a "Chlorine Free Campaign" calling for a worldwide ban on chlorine, and there has been a strong anti-chlorine sentiment in the U.S. Environmental Protection Agency (EPA) and the U.S. Congress.[20]

What You Need to Know About the Chlorine in Sucralose

According to Splenda.com, we shouldn't worry about the chlorine in sucralose, as it is a safe and natural part of our food supply.

> Chlorine is present naturally in many of the foods and beverages that we eat and drink every day ranging from lettuce, mushrooms and table salt.[21]

But if chlorine is toxic, how can this be?

It is because there is no chlorine in food and table salt. There is chloride however. The difference between chloride and chlorine is like the difference between Dr. Jekyl and Mr. Hyde.

As stated before, chlorine is a highly reactive element which does not exist by itself in nature but only in combination with other elements (usually sodium or potassium).[22] This is because when chlorine reacts with sodium, for example, the sodium transfers an electron to the chlorine atom resulting in a positively charged sodium ion and a negatively charged chloride ion. These oppositely charged ions attract which forms a stable *ionic bond*. Ionic compounds such as salt, have the following properties:

- they tend to form crystalline solids

- they dissolve in water

- they have high melting temperatures.[23]

Chloride exists mainly in the form of salt. It is the main negative ion found in the ocean; it is present in the body fluids of animals; it is essential for life and is completely non-toxic, and this is why salt is safe to eat.[24]

We know that Splenda is completely different from salt because salt has a stable ionic bond between sodium and chloride in salt, and there are no carbon atoms in salt. On the other hand, the manufacturing of Splenda involves the artificial replacement of hydrogen atoms in sugar with chlorine atoms and forces the chlorine atoms to form a covalent bond with carbon. Molecules which contain bonds between chlorine and carbons are called *chlorocarbons* or *organochlorines*. As Dr. James Bowen, a physician and biochemist, writes, the covalent bond between chlorine and carbon is what makes chlorocarbons harmful to life:

Unlike sodium chloride, chlorocarbons are never nutritionally compatible with our metabolic processes and are wholly incompatible with normal human metabolic functioning. When chlorine is chemically reacted into carbon-structured organic compounds to make chlorocarbons, the carbon and chlorine atoms bind to each other by mutually sharing electrons in their outer shells. This arrangement adversely affects human metabolism because our mitochondrial and cellular enzyme systems are designed to completely utilize organic molecules containing carbon, hydrogen, oxygen, nitrogen, and other compatible nutritional elements. By this process chlorocarbons such as sucralose deliver chlorine directly into our cells through normal metabolization. This makes them effective insecticides . . .

Any chlorocarbons not directly excreted from the body intact can cause immense damage to the processes of human metabolism and, eventually, our internal organs. The liver is a detoxification organ which deals with ingested poisons. Chlorocarbons damage the hepatocytes, the liver's metabolic cells, and destroy them.[25]

When you add chlorine to carbon-containing compounds to form organochlorines, they have the potential to be converted into a toxic pesticide, one that can cause you severe and permanent neurologic and immune dysfunctions, or cause cancer. Organochlorines as a group are mainly used as pesticides, such as DDT, dieldrin, aldrin, lindane, chlordane, and heptachlor. Remember that sucralose was also discovered while trying to create a new insecticide. Other organochlorines, like carbon tetrachloride and trichloroethylene, are used as solvents. Freon refrigerants are hydrocarbons that have been both chlorinated and fluorinated (chlorofluorocarbons, or CFC's—well known for causing depletion of the ozone layer).

Organochlorines have come under considerable scrutiny because of their persistence in the environment and the human body. Notorious chlorinated compounds include "Agent Orange," where dioxin is the chlorinated culprit, and polychlorinated biphenyls (PCBs). PCBs were available from 1929 to 1975 and were used as transformer and electrical equipment.

PCBs have consistently been associated with both cancer and abnormalities within the reproductive, immune, and nervous systems. The studies that document these associations, if they were stacked on the floor, would be far taller than you.

Organochlorines are fat-soluble by definition, although their solubility can vary considerably. Fat-soluble substances tend to accumulate in organ tissues that are high in fat, such as your brain. And even worse—they are permanently stored there.[26]

The bioaccumulation of chlorinated compounds in your fat is a major concern, because once a fat cell is made in your body, it's typically there for the rest of your life. Your fat cells can shrink and expand as you lose or gain weight, but they and the toxins they contain will remain unless they are somehow detoxified.

Organochlorine toxicity mainly affects your brain, heart, and lungs. The symptoms are varied and depend upon the length of exposure.[27] Fat-soluble compounds like organochlorines also often do not decay in the environment.[28] One reason DDT is so devastating is that it stays in the food chain for many years, causing genetic mutations in many animals that come in contact with it. This is why many toxic organochlorines, such as DDT, have been banned in the United States and worldwide. But there are hundreds of types of organochlorines used. An estimated three million cases of severe pesticide poisoning and 220,000 deaths occur each year due to organochlorine pesticide use.[29]

More Sweet, Devious Deception

In an effort to disassociate itself from the ominous organochlorine group of chemicals, McNeil Nutritionals has conveniently created out of thin air their own chemical group category name for sucralose. Their official product literature states that sucralose is not an organochlorine, but rather a "chloro-carbohydrate."

You might wonder if this chemical class exists for any other substances. Well no, it doesn't. I believe they made up the new term to help them avoid any associations with the other notorious chlorinated compounds that have such a menacing history.

The simple fact is that sucralose is indeed a organochlorine, because it is a carbon and hydrogen molecule with attached chlorine atoms.

Because organochlorines as a class are fat-soluble, sucralose should also be fat-soluble. However, McNeil states that sucralose is somehow the exception to the rule and is "almost insoluble in fat."[30]

Note the word "almost," which means that there is at least some fat solubility. However, regardless of the degree of water or fat solubility and the associated possibility of chronic toxicity, organochlorines don't have to be fat soluble to cause harm as they can cause significant damage to the body immediately upon contact.

Organochlorine Toxicity

The following is a list of the more common symptoms of organochlorine toxicity. You will notice some of many of these symptoms in the case studies in this chapter of people who have had reactions to sucralose:

Short-Term Exposure: agitation, lethargy, seizures, hallucinations, respiratory complaints, *irregular heartbeat, cough,* shortness of breath, *nausea,* vomiting, *diarrhea, abdominal pain, skin rashes, headaches, dizziness, paralysis* of the face, tongue, and extremities, respiratory failure, ear, nose, and throat irritation, blurred vision, pulmonary edema (water in the lungs).

Long-Term Exposure: lack of appetite, liver and kidney damage, central nervous system disturbances (dizziness, hallucinations, *headaches,* coma, tremors, etc.), *skin irritation.*

NAME OF ORGANOCHLORINE	PURPOSE	SAFETY RECORD
DDT	Insecticide	Banned in North America due to severe toxicity
Dicofol	Insecticide	Banned in many countries due to environmental toxicity[31]
Methoxychlor	Insecticide	Has been shown to be neurotoxic and endocrine toxic in high doses[32]
Chlorobenzilate	Insecticide	Banned in the United States due to studies showing increased cancer in mice[33]
Aldrin and Dieldrin	Pesticides for crops and for termites	Banned by the EPA in 1974 due to harm to environment and human health except for termite control
Chlordane	Insecticide	Banned in 1988 due to harm to humans and the environment[34]
Trans-Nonachlor	Insecticide	Banned after 1988 due to cancer risk

Heptachlor epoxide	Insecticide for cotton and termites	Liver damage, excitability, and decreases in fertility, possible human carcinogen[35]
PCBs	Used as electrical insulators and heat agents	Banned in many countries due to its inability to break down in the environment and food chain
Pentachlorophenol (PCP) and tetrachlorophenol (TCP)	Insecticide for wood preservation	Skin penetration has caused a 60% death rate[36]
Hexachlorobenzene (HCB)	Fungicide and pesticide for grain. Also used in tire manufacturing	Banned in 1970s as a pesticide due to environmental toxicity. Harms the endocrine system (hormones)[37]
Dioxins PCDDs and PCDFs (210 kinds)	By-products of other chemicals (e.g. pesticides and wood preservatives)	Increases cancer risk, diabetes, liver and heart diseases, skin problems[38]
Vinyl chloride and PVC	Used to manufacture plastics, building materials, toys	Linked to cancer, birth defects, damage to the liver, lungs, blood, nervous system[39]
Phosgene	Chemical warfare, manufacturing	Lethal respiratory poison
Mustard gas	Chemical warfare	Lethal respiratory poison
Chloroform	Originally used as an anesthetic, Solvents	Due to carcinogenicity, it has been banned as an anesthetic and has fallen out of favor as a solvent
Dichloromethane	Solvents	Chronic exposure may be carcinogenic
Dichloroethene	Solvents	Has caused nervous system disorders, liver and kidney diseases, and lung problems in humans[40]

Trichloroethane	Solvents	Banned in 2002 for destroying the ozone layer, high levels may cause unconsciousness and death[41]
Sucralose/Splenda	Food sweetener	The only organochlorine ever used for human consumption[42]

CINDY'S STORY

Two years ago, Cindy began drinking fruit smoothies sweetened with sucralose on a daily basis. Not long afterward, she was diagnosed with Bell's Palsy—a twitching or paralysis of the face—which affected her on the right side. One week after that, she was diagnosed with trigeminal neuralgia when she began experiencing excruciating pain in the same areas affected by the palsy. Cindy continued drinking her smoothies, never suspecting it could be playing a role in her symptoms.

Eight months later she began to experience mild seizures, during which she lost all ability to communicate and was completely disoriented. She realized that she had similar symptoms in the past when she ate aspartame, which she now avoided.

Finally deciding to take it upon herself to investigate the cause of her symptoms, Cindy eventually found Mercola.com and realized the possibility that her diet might be causing the problem.

One week after halting all consumption of her sucralose smoothies, Cindy's condition began to improve. Cindy is now happy to report that she is symptom-free and staying away from sucralose for good.

Incredibly Effective Deceptive Marketing Campaign

McNeil has been enormously successful in marketing Splenda. They have convinced nearly half of U.S consumers that sucralose is actually a natural product. In April of 2004, the Center for Science in the Public

Interest (CSPI) conducted a national Internet Survey that included 426 people who consume sucralose- or Splenda-containing products. Only 57 percent of Splenda users correctly identified it as an artificial sweetener. Forty-three percent of consumers believe that it's a natural product.[43]

Just 8 percent were able to correctly identify the fact that sucralose is made from chlorine as well as sugar. Only this small percentage knew they were consuming a chemical that no natural sugar product contains. Clearly, McNeil has been very effective in concealing this fact.

Recently, the Order of Professional Dieticians of Quebec (OPDQ), a professional group of nutritionists in Canada, awarded McNeil and Johnson & Johnson the 2005 Rotten Apple award. The Rotten Apple award is given to the food company that causes the most confusion about the concept of a health food or the nutritional value of a product. OPDQ chose Johnson & Johnson's "Dance of the Splenda Plum Fairy" print advertisement, because it claims that the chemical sweetener can be used "everywhere you use sugar" and is "an excellent reason to spoil your loved ones." The ad features a young child eating cookies.

OPDQ stated that this ad won the award "for marketing that evokes the idea that their product (an artificial sugar substitute) can be used everywhere sugar can be used and can be given to children without limitation. The ads also maintain it has the taste of sugar."[44]

Samantha Heller, MS, RD, speaks clearly of the true nature of Splenda in a WebMD article when she says, "Saying Splenda is made from sugar is like taking the round wheels off a car and putting on square wheels. Is it still a car? Yes. But can it still perform like a car? No. And what's more we don't know what's going to happen when people try to drive that car cross country."[45]

Sweet Deception In Sucralose's Name

The typical names assigned to sugars end in the suffix "-ose." Examples of this are sucrose, glucose, fructose, dextrose, etc. Understanding this nomenclature is one of the ways that you can begin to decipher the list of ingredients on a food label. You can be alerted to any hidden sources of sugar that might be present in the food.

This naming scheme has led well-educated, health-conscious consumers and health care professionals, who carefully look at labels before purchasing their food item, to pick up a product that contains sucralose (easily mistaken for the word *sucrose*), read the ingredients, and conclude that the product does not contain any artificial chemicals that could possibly harm them.

This is an absolutely brilliant marketing strategy for McNeil. By a simple naming sleight of hand, they have been able to convince nearly everyone that they are consuming a natural sugar.

Unfortunately this brilliance only serves McNeil, not you.

During the final push for FDA approval, several groups, including consumer advocacy groups, attempted to dispute the name of sucralose on the grounds that it would confuse consumers. It was suggested that the final product be called "trichlorogalactosucrose," which more appropriately describes its chemical structure and nature. Although this name still ends in an "-ose," at least it more clearly represents the fact that sucralose is in no way a simple sugar similar to sucrose or glucose, as its name currently implies, but is in fact a complex chlorinated artificial chemical.

The FDA and McNeil Nutritionals ignored the requests and plowed forward with the misleading name. One of the justifications was that it was already regulated under the name "sucralose" in Canada and Australia (a situation they had actively lobbied for), so therefore it would be appropriate to make it "consistent" with other English speaking countries.

The FDA also argued in their final rule that precise chemical names are difficult for people to understand. They pointed out that other artificial sweeteners such as aspartame do not use their chemical names, and there has been no confusion from that.[46]

It defies all common sense that the FDA could argue that because the name "aspartame" has never been confused with "sucrose," that "sucralose" won't be confused with "sucrose." But as we can see, truth and logic are not the deciding factors when it comes to FDA approval.

Fighting Back

Because McNeil pitches Splenda as a "natural healthy product," many health food stores carry it in their sweetener section. Recently, though, a number of health food store owners have begun to understand its synthetic and potentially harmful nature, and are pulling it off their shelves. Whole Foods Markets, one of the nation's largest health food store chains, has decided not to carry Splenda- or sucralose-containing foods on the following premise:

> Although sucralose is "derived from sugar," it is also a highly processed additive created by the manipulation of molecules. Sucralose does not fit within the Whole Foods standard of being minimally processed. Finally, despite its derivation from plain sugar (a feature the manufacturer repeatedly emphasizes), sucralose is an artificial sweetener. Historically, our company has avoided selling non-nutritive artificial sweeteners because they are not in accordance with our philosophy of promoting "real" food.[47]

Lawsuits Against Splenda

As a result of McNeil's advertising claims, they are being sued by a number of people, social interest groups, and organizations, including some from the sugar industry. In December of 2004, the Sugar Association filed suit against McNeil for deceptive advertising over that famous "made from sugar, so it tastes like sugar" slogan. Although they admittedly have a self interest in this case, I believe the Sugar Association is spot-on in their argument; consumers are being misled into thinking that Splenda is natural, when it is not natural at all.[48]

In addition to being sued by the sugar industry, a lawsuit has been filed against McNeil by Merisant Co., the makers of the aspartame-based Equal. They, too, are criticizing McNeil and trying to make them stop associating their product so closely with sugar.

McNeil subsequently sued the Sugar Association in February 2005 for libel in connection with the Web site TruthAboutSplenda.com, but on March 29, 2006, their lawsuit against the Sugar Association was dismissed; according to a federal court in Wilmington, Delaware, McNeil had "no right to maintain an independent action."[49]

There is a growing list of consumer groups who are petitioning against

Splenda's misleading advertising, including the California Alliance for Consumer Protection, Organic Consumers Association, the Center for Science in the Public Interest, Florida Consumer Action Network, www.TruthAboutSplenda.com, NYPIRG, Texas Consumer Association and Citizens For Health.[50]

MICHELLE'S STORY

Michelle was invited over to her friend's house for coffee. She asked for sugar in her coffee, but her friend only had Splenda® No Calorie Sweetener on hand, so she used that for the first time. After only a few sips, she began to feel a severe tingling sensation in the back of her neck. Soon she began to feel panicked and anxious. Her heart raced. Then her throat began to swell shut, and her limbs went numb.

Michelle was quickly taken to the emergency room. She had no idea what had caused the attack. It wasn't until she was answering a doctor's questions in the ER that she realized that moments before the attack, she had consumed Splenda for the first time.

It took Michelle days to fully recover from her symptoms. She's avoided Splenda ever since and has never had another allergic reaction.

The Sucralose Studies

To research this book, I carefully plodded through the two-foot stack of documents and memorandums that were involved in the FDA final ruling for the approval of sucralose as a food additive.

There are only six published human studies on sucralose. One of these is a case report of a migraine patient taking sucralose, so this does not really qualify as a study, leaving only five. The longest sucralose was studied in the published human trials was thirteen weeks. However, McNeil submitted unpublished research to the FDA that studied humans taking sucralose for a total of six months. But it is important to note that these studies only focused on the effect of sucralose on blood sugar in diabetics and did not focus on overall safety.

We are aware of only three long-term trials in animals: one study using

104 mice[51] and one using 104 rats over a two year period, and a twelve-month oral toxicity study in dogs.[52]

The FDA Final Rule concluded that "the available data and information submitted in a food additive petition must establish, to a reasonable certainty, that the food additive is not harmful under the intended conditions of use."

However, after carefully reviewing the evidence, I have reached a different conclusion: that there are simply no long-term safety trials done on *any* humans, none, nada, zero, zip, nothing but animal studies to assure you that using this sweetener for years will not cause you any serious health problems.

McNeil assures you of Splenda's safety by stating on their Web site that "the safety of sucralose is well documented in more than 100 scientific studies conducted over a 20-year period."

Unfortunately, not all of these studies are published for the public to review. According to the National Library of Medicine, as of early August 2006, only eighty-four scientific research articles on sucralose had been published. You can view the actual list of these studies at www.sweet deception.com/studies.

Eighty-four studies still sounds like quite a few . . . until you look at them more carefully and you discover that nearly 80 percent of the published studies had absolutely nothing to do with independently evaluating sucralose safety in animals or humans. There were more published studies examining whether or not it caused dental decay than whether or not it was safe to consume.

PUBLISHED STUDIES INDEX MEDICUS	# OF STUDIES
Measurements of sucralose (e.g., to measure intestinal permeability)	28
Dental decay	17
Artificial sweetener taste preferences in animals	12
Reviews of sucralose studies	12
Safety studies in animals (10 published in one issue of one journal)	10
Safety studies in humans	5
Total (As of July 5, 2006)	84

So out of eighty-four published studies, *only fifteen* were done on animals or humans to evaluate the safety of sucralose. Of those, only five were human trials.

Most of the information that McNeil uses to justify sucralose's approval was based on unpublished studies that were privately submitted to the FDA and are not available for public review. Why aren't these studies available to the public? Can we trust the FDA's decision to approve sucralose, just as they approved aspartame?

Does This Make Any Sense?

In those five published human safety trials, sucralose was only tested on approximately 191 people total. In my research for this book, I have received more anecdotal case reports from people who have experienced adverse reactions to sucralose than there are people sucralose was formally tested on.[53]

Something is seriously wrong here.

It is also important to understand that only two of the human trials were conducted and published before the FDA granted approval for sucralose to be used as a "general purpose" sweetener in 1999. The FDA determined sucralose to be safe for human consumption based primarily on animal studies. Unfortunately, there is a great deal of variation between humans and the different animal species in terms of how they react to chemical compounds, including sucralose.

The longest human toxicity trial was a mere thirteen weeks—hardly long enough when you consider that the typical consumer will use sucralose over the course of a lifetime. The conclusion that sucralose is safe is based on seriously inadequate human safety studies. But this premature assessment has been used to give the green light for people to use as much sucralose as their heart's, desire.

Who's Doing All This Research?

There appears to be a bit of bias when it comes to the science behind sucralose. We understand that Tate & Lyle and McNeil have commissioned or performed over 76 percent of the published studies that have been conducted on sucralose safety, and as many as 98 percent of the total published and unpublished safety studies used by the FDA during Splenda's approval. This calculation was performed on the assumption that McNeil submitted at least 171 studies to the FDA. We did not see all the studies, but McNeil used sequential numbering on all the studies submitted and the highest number we saw was 171. Eighty-four studies were also published in *Medline*.

Of the fifteen published animal and human safety studies, thirteen were directly funded by the manufacturer. There are only two independent human studies that address sucralose safety—which are poorly designed and are therefore, in my opinion, inconclusive.[54]

Remember that an analysis of 166 articles on aspartame found that 100 percent of the 74 studies financed by the industry attested to aspartame's safety. However, of the 92 independently funded articles, 91 percent identified adverse health effects.[55] So it is important to pay careful attention to who is funding the sucralose studies, as sucralose may follow a similar pattern.

When a pharmaceutical company develops a new drug, they frequently run a handful of trials themselves, both animal and human. This makes sense, because they are testing a product to see if it even works for the intended purpose for which it is prescribed.

But when practically all studies conducted are by the manufacturer of a product, there is, in my view, clearly a case of obvious bias and a potential for a profoundly serious conflict of interest. There is absolutely no incentive for the researchers to find anything but data that would support the approval of their own product. There are strong incentives to only report the positive studies.

A far better system, which could drastically reduce the influence of potential conflicts of interest, would be for the manufacturers to pay a fee to the FDA, which could hire out testing by an anonymous independent lab and use that unbiased data for approval.

Just Who Was Tested to Prove that Sucralose Was Safe?

Study populations must be a valid sample of the group potentially affected. Sucralose will be eaten by humans; we are not feeding it to our pet dogs, rabbits, cats, or rats.

Sound science would dictate that a product should be proven safe in all genders, ages, and groups of a human population. We can't assume that sucralose is good for women, children, pregnant women, the ill, and the elderly (who, combined, make up the world's population) in the absence of any data confirming this. The vast majority of test subjects in the few human studies are middle-aged men. And the bulk of the very limited data that supports the assertion that sucralose is safe is based on animal studies.

Splenda has never been tested in the majority of people that are using it.

Human studies performed on drugs are tested on thousands to hundreds of thousands of individuals. Even then, after a drug passes a clinical trial, it is often later taken off the market after fatal complications are identified that did not show up in the initial studies. In half of the human trials of sucralose, there were less than 30 individuals tested. The largest published human sucralose trial only studied 128 individuals for three months. This is normally considered a *small* study population. These numbers are hardly consistent with scientific validity, nor do they justify allowing sucralose to be consumed by hundreds of millions of people. In an internal 1994 memorandum, FDA pharmacologist William Roth, PhD, voiced his concerns about the paltry number of human studies McNeil submitted for sucralose approval: "It should be kept in mind that we have seen metabolic data only for a very small number of humans, and only for one sex."[56]

TONI AND CHUCK'S STORY

A little over a year ago, Toni and Chuck began drinking diet soda sweetened with sucralose. Right away, Toni developed a terrible rash on her face and neck and felt very fatigued. Meanwhile, Chuck developed aches and pains in his joints and had daily bouts of nausea and bloating.

At first, Toni and Chuck attributed all of their problems to things like changes in the weather, arthritis, allergies, or old age. But when their symptoms persisted for more than a year, they began to think something was seriously wrong. Then one day, while doing some research on the Internet, Toni discovered the various articles and testimonials about the potential dangers of sucralose on my Web site, Mercola.com.[57]

They immediately stopped all intake of Splenda, and they've already begun noticing a decrease in their symptoms. After enduring over a year of misery, Toni's rash is going away, and she feels her energy coming back, and Chuck's nausea has subsided.

Is Sucralose Digested Or Not?

Normally, when you ingest an organochlorine, it is absorbed through your colon and enters your bloodstream, and your liver then attempts to detoxify this foreign chemical by combining it with glucuronic acid (a process called glucuronidation) to make it more water soluble so it can be carried out of your body via the urine or bile. If your detoxification mechanisms are overwhelmed by a high toxic load, or if they are impaired due to poor health, your body will not be able to effectively eliminate organochlorines and you will store them in your fat cells, where they will continue to poison you indefinitely.

This is why the question of what happens to sucralose in your body is such a crucial one and is clearly the primary reason McNeil strongly insists that sucralose is different from all the other organochlorines, and is instead safely excreted from the body mostly unchanged. Let's examine the statements made by McNeil about absorption, excretion, metabolism, and distribution one-by-one.

Absorption of Sucralose

The Health Professionals section of the Splenda.com Web site has this to say about the absorption of sucralose:

Absorption

The majority (about 85 percent) of consumed sucralose is not absorbed and passes through the gastrointestinal tract unchanged. Approximately 15 percent of ingested sucralose is passively absorbed, which is related to the fact that sucralose is a very small, very water soluble molecule.[58]

Likewise, the FDA final ruling on sucralose concluded that sucralose is "poorly absorbed" following ingestion.

It sounds very reassuring. Eating sucralose is like drinking a glass of water; it just passes right though, no problems.

However, that isn't exactly the case.

To start with, the 15 percent number is an imprecise "average" absorption rate, because people vary widely in their absorption abilities. The range for humans has been estimated to be 11–27 percent, according to the FDA review of studies. An absorption rate of 27 percent is not what I call "poorly absorbed." This is almost one-third. But even the range of 11–27 percent is very imprecise; most of the absorption and metabolism data provided to the FDA for sucralose approval was done on animals, which, according to the FDA final ruling, were used to extrapolate the safety in humans.[59] The problem with this is there is a great deal of variation of absorption and metabolism among different species.

ESTIMATION OF ORAL SUCRALOSE ABSORPTION

	McNeil Estimates[60]	FDA Estimates[61]
Rat	10%	5%
Man	15%	11–27%
Rabbit	20%	20–33%
Mouse	30%	20–33%
Dog	35%	33–36%

Given that each species has such different absorption rates and digestive capacities, it seems the only truly reliable absorption and metabolism studies would be those done on humans.

And yet, there is only one published study on absorption and metabolism in humans, and this study looked at a *single dose* of sucralose given to only *eight healthy young men*. They absorbed from as little as 9 percent to as much as 22 percent of their dose of sucralose.[62]

There were eight other human studies studying metabolism and pharmacokinetics submitted to the FDA, but these were not published, so we do not have access to them.

So the human absorption rates are based on healthy male subjects. Unfortunately, we have no data on absorption rates in other populations such as infants, children, pregnant women, the elderly, and those with disease conditions such as inflammatory bowel disease. Inflammatory bowel disease is an important issue; if you are a person who suffers from any digestive system problems such as irritable bowel, diarrhea, or inflammatory bowel disease, you have a far higher likelihood of sucralose passing from your digestive system rapidly into your bloodstream. In fact, researchers are now using radio-labeled sucralose to identify individuals who have "Leaky Gut Syndrome."[63]

Unfortunately, most people nowadays have a leaky gut to some extent, because there are so many products in our culture that cause intestinal inflammation such as alcohol, caffeine, processed food, sugar, non steroidal anti-inflammatory drugs "NSAIDs", birth control pills, and prednisone. Therefore, most of the population is at risk for absorbing sucralose at levels at the upper ranges of 27 percent or more.

In summary, sucralose absorption has not been adequately tested in a variety of populations, or for long periods of time. However, the bigger question is, what happens once sucralose enters your bloodstream?

Distribution of Sucralose In Your Body

The Splenda.com Web site has this to say about the distribution of sucralose:

Distribution

Because it is highly water soluble, absorbed sucralose is distributed to essentially all tissues. Sucralose is not lipophilic and does not bioaccumulate.[64]

If it is true that sucralose is water soluble and does not bioaccumulate accumulate in the tissues), as McNeil emphasizes repeatedly, it must be the rare exception to the rule that organochlorides are fat-soluble, and therefore will build up in the body tissues.

Should we take McNeil's word for it?

Not so fast. There are a few concerns about this issue. First of all, sucralose is somewhat soluble in ethyl acetate.[65] Ethyl acetate is used as a solvent for fat-soluble substances, so this may indicate that sucralose is at least slightly fat soluble.

Second, the human and animal studies on sucralose metabolism state that the metabolites (digestive breakdown products) of sucralose are *glucuronide* conjugates of sucralose. Glucuronidation, as you might recall, is the process in which your liver combines glucuronic acid with potentially *toxic, fat-soluble substances* to make them more water-soluble for subsequent elimination into your urine or bile.[66]

According to Shane Ellison, a pharmaceutical chemist, and author of *Health Myths Exposed,*

> The fact that sucralose undergoes glucuronidation is prima facie evidence that at least a portion of the sucralose molecule or its metabolites are fat soluble. The purpose of glucuronidation is to make substances water soluble and if sucralose were entirely water soluble, the glucuronidation detox pathway would not be necessary.

To definitively prove that sucralose is not fat soluble, there should be an analysis of fat samples of humans after long-term exposure, but this has not been reported and, to the best of our knowledge, has not been done.

Prior to the FDA Final Ruling that concluded that sucralose was safe, Dr. William Roth, a pharmacologist at the FDA, stated in a FDA memo that the lack of distribution data made it impossible to determine that sucralose was safe for humans and unborn fetuses:

> Questions raised in an earlier review about . . . systemic exposure in general have yet to be answered with a good study design and hard experimental data. Without this information . . . it would be difficult to have much confidence in any extrapolations made to human systemic exposure, placental transfer, or exposure to the fetus . . . Since the quality of the data available for tissue distribution in the rat is low, and no information is available for other species, no reliable estimates can be made of the levels of sucralose that might be achieved in the tissues of humans consuming sucralose.[67]

Basically, we believe there is simply not enough data to truly understand how, or to what extent, sucralose is distributed in your body. It appears that both the FDA and McNeil expect you to trust that when sucralose, originally discovered in the search for new insecticides, is distributed to your blood, brain, heart, kidneys, lungs, intestines, and to your unborn fetus, there's no need to be concerned as long as you do not eat more than the FDA acceptable daily limit.

ANGELA'S STORY

Angela was watching her carbs, and was thrilled to find the wide variety of low-carb foods available at her local health food story. Most of them were sweetened with sucralose.

About a week after she started eating them, she developed excessive gas, bloating, and some diarrhea. At first, she dismissed the symptoms, thinking they were probably a flare-up of her Irritable Bowel Syndrome. But a few months later, she began to experience excruciating stomach spasms. They would last for about ten of fifteen minutes, and then vanish, only to recur later.

The pain was intense. Her heart rate shot up into the 150s. On one occasion, she went to the ER, where she was given morphine for the pain.

One day, she heard that other people were having intestinal problems related to sucralose. Curious, she cut the low-carb foods out of her diet. Several months passed without any stomach spasms. As a test, she introduced it back into her diet by adding Splenda to her morning coffee. The bloating immediately returned, and within about two weeks, so did the stomach spasms.

She no longer uses any artificial sweeteners and carefully reads ingredient labels for sucralose. Her symptoms have not returned.

Elimination of Sucralose

According to Splenda.com, "Most ingested sucralose is eliminated unchanged in the stool with no *gastrointestinal effects.*"[68]

However, studies have shown gastrointestinal tract disturbances[69] and, loose stools[70] in animals fed sucralose, and we have many testimonials from people, like Angela, who experienced gastrointestinal effects such as bloating, cramping, diarrhea, and vomiting after using sucralose.

Splenda.com also states:

In *all* species tested, including humans, over 95 percent of the consumed dose is excreted either in the feces (unabsorbed fraction) or urine (absorbed fraction) as unchanged sucralose. Of the small amount of sucralose that crosses into the bloodstream, which is excreted largely as unchanged sucralose . . . *all* is eliminated via the urine . . ."[71]

This paragraph essentially states that all species eliminate *100 percent* of sucralose from their body. But study findings directly contradict this. One rabbit study showed only 80 percent elimination by the study's end.[72]

The FDA Final Rule cited the following three concerns of the legal firm Malkin regarding the possibility of sucralose bioaccumulation:

1. There is a potential for sucralose to accumulate in the fetus, because of its extremely slow elimination from fetal tissue.

2. Sucralose has a half-life of twenty-four hours before excretion is "indicative of the potential for sucralose to accumulate in the body of consumers."

3. Human studies showed that 4–7 percent of the sucralose was not excreted five days after a single dosing. [Authors note: Actually the study of eight men showed up to 12 percent] and dog studies showed 20 percent of the sucralose remained in the body four days after dosing, which "represents either potential bioaccumulation, extensive in vivo dechlorination, or both."

If up to 12 percent remains in the body, where does it go and what does it do? Is it stored in the cells, or the fat? If up to 12 percent stays in your body every time sucralose is consumed, how much sucralose would accumulate if you consume sucralose every day as so many people do? Does it remain in your body indefinitely?

Let me ask you this: if I handed you a bottle and said, "Here, drink this sweetened chlorinated solution. Don't worry, its safe, because only 12 percent of it will stay in your body"—would you drink it?

The FDA's response to Malkin's concerns is paraphrased as follows:

1. There is not enough pharmacokinetic data to show whether or not there was bioaccumulation of sucralose.

2. But because it is mostly water soluble, it does not have a high potential for bioaccumulation.

3. In addition, sucralose is poorly absorbed from the gut in humans (11 to 27 percent).

4. Finally, there is little or no evidence of direct tissue toxicity from sucralose in the mouse, rat, and dog, even when administered at high doses for one to two years which is more important than bioaccumulation.

Half of the justification as to why the FDA concluded that this was not a significant issue was due to insufficient data and their reliance on sucralose's poor absorption. However, as we have previously shown, there seems to be a serious question as to the reliability of this data with respect to its generalization to the entire human population.

It would seem that there is ample justification to disagree with the FDA's conclusions, as there are numerous red flags in the areas of absorption, distribution, excretion, and metabolism, and only a handful of human studies to prove safety, all of which are limited by sample size, methodology. and duration.

Metabolism of Sucralose

The purpose of digestion is for your body to metabolize (break down) food into its smallest components, so that they can be absorbed through your intestines and into your bloodstream, where the nutrients can enter your cells. The reason that the metabolism of sucralose is a key issue is that once the sucralose molecule is broken down into smaller fragments, it becomes much more difficult to know the effect each fragment (metabolite) has on the body. And in the case of sucralose, the FDA has stated that there may be at least twenty-one possible constituents consisting of two hydrolysis products, fourteen byproduct chlorinated compounds and five intermediates.[73]

Furthermore, the more your body metabolizes sucralose, the more likely that potentially toxic and unknown chlorinated molecules may be liberated from the sucralose molecule.

To allay your fears of such an alarming scenario, McNeil assures us at Splenda.com that the metabolism of sucralose is completely harmless:

Distribution

Sucralose is not recognized by the body as a carbohydrate—it is not broken down for energy and provides no calories. Approximately 2 percent of ingested sucralose is biotransformed into toxicologically insignificant components and excreted in the urine. Sucralose does not bind to blood or other proteins. There is also no dechlorination or breakdown of the molecule to its component monosaccharide-like derivatives.[74]

Despite the fact that McNeil states there is "no breakdown of the sucralose molecule" into its "component monosaccharide-like derivatives," this once again directly contradicts the documents they submitted to the FDA, which state:

... These studies pointed to the fact that sucralose, a disaccharide, will hydrolyze to its constituent monosaccharides during both wet and dry storage.[75]

Hydrolysis is the decomposition of a chemical compound by reaction with water. According to the FDA Final Rule, "Hydrolysis of sucralose can occur under conditions of prolonged storage at elevated temperatures in highly acidic aqueous food products." The legal firm Malkin stated that in acidic drinks, such as carbonated soft drinks, sucralose concentrations decrease by 4–20 percent after six months of storage, which may expose humans to higher levels than the acceptable daily intake for these hydrolysis products.

Both the Scientific Committee for Food, the regulatory body which issues approval for the sale of sweeteners in Europe, and the Center for Science in the Public Interest have expressed concern about the hydrolysis products in sucralose and would like more safety data on the mutagenic properties. Trace amounts of 1,6-chlorofructose are sometimes found in canned drinks left to stand for several months.[76] In the study of sucralose metabolism, McNeil has identified at least two major hydrolysis products of sucralose: 1,6-dichloro-1,6-dideoxyfructose (1,6-DCF) and 4- chloro-4-deoxygalactose (4-CG).[77]

McNeil has performed numerous studies on these breakdown products, because other chlorosugars like 6-chloro-6-deoxy-glucose (6-CG) have been shown to cause infertility and brain damage in animals.[78] Furthermore, McNeil admits that sucralose has the theoretical potential to also break down into the highly toxic chlorosugar 6-GC, but they contend that the amount would be so small it that would be negligible.[79] Even if the potential amount is "negligible," I'd prefer my ingestion of potentially toxic chlorosugars be "zero."

Regardless of whether or not sucralose turns into 6-CG, studies show that the digestion products of sucralose (1,6-DCF and/or 4-CG) can cause:[80]

- Liver toxicity (E136)

- Depletion of glutathione (your ability to detoxify) (E136)

- Weak mutagenic (causing genetic changes) activity[81]

- Binding to the DNA of the liver and small intestine two hours after ingestion[82] (E148)

- Enlarged livers in rat fetuses even at the lowest possible dose[83] (E054)

- Low-birth weight in rat offspring[84] (E052)

- Maternal and fetal toxicity[85] (E032)

McNeil's position is that the FDA Final Rule states that the no-observed effect level for the hydrolysis products is tens of thousands of times higher than the estimated daily intake (EDI) and therefore allows an adequate safety margin for the hydrolysis products.

As if the questionable toxic breakdown products 1,6-DCF and 4-CG weren't bad enough, there are further references to 1,6-DCF converting to a molecule 6-chlorofructose, which caused paralysis in mice after only eight days of treatment.[86]

The Metabolism section of Splenda.com also states: "There is also no dechlorination . . . ," meaning that the chlorine in Splenda is not released from the molecule. But if this is indeed true, then why did McNeil submit a study to the FDA entitled: "1 ,6-dichloro–1 ,6-dideoxyfructose: Metabolism And *Dechlorination* in the Rat," which documented how the chlorine atoms came off the sucralose molecule during metabolism?[87]

Furthermore, according to an FDA memo from James Griffiths, PhD, toxicologist for the FDA,[88] "The Splenda metabolite DCF has been shown in past studies[89] to *spontaneously dechlorinate* in vitro [outside the living organism], though at a very slow rate. The rapid in vivo [in the living organism] dechlorination is cell-mediated, and involves . . . dechlorination at the C-1 position in liver and RBCs." So it seems that sucralose does indeed dechlorinate. Are you beginning to notice a pattern here? Isn't it curious that so much of the documentation McNeil submitted to the FDA says the opposite of what McNeil is telling the public? Hydrolysis of sucralose may or may not occur depending on the storage conditions. What does occur every time sucralose is ingested is the breakdown into smaller metabolites. McNeil approximates that only 2 percent of the sucralose is broken down, but once again, the actual data found in the one human trial of eight men actually showed a range of 1–5 percent. There were no comments in this study about the possible significance, or toxicity, of these metabolites.[90]

ANN'S STORY

Fifteen months ago, Ann started a low-carb diet. She began to consume more and more of the increasingly popular "low-carb friendly" food items. Shortly thereafter, Ann began to break out in a rash on her neck, which quickly spread. Soon her scalp and back were so itchy that she felt like an animal infested with fleas. She simply could not stop scratching.

Desperate, Ann began eliminating commonly allergenic foods like nuts and eggs from her diet, hoping the horrible rash was due to an allergic reaction. While cutting these foods out, she also increased her consumption of processed foods, like ice cream and candy, sweetened with sucralose. Since Ann loved these foods, she decided that she would eliminate them only if everything else failed.

Everything else did. As a last-ditch effort, Ann finally got on the Internet to try and find out if sucralose could be the culprit. She was shocked to discover the horror stories from people who had suffered from the exact same symptoms she had. Ann even discovered she was suffering from other symptoms she hadn't connected with the rash at all such as loose stools.

Ann stopped eating all sucralose products immediately, and within a week, her rash, itching, and loose stools disappeared completely.

Interestingly, the FDA in its final ruling did not at all dispute any of the digestion issues we've covered in these past few sections and stated the available pharmacokinetic data *did not allow them to draw definitive conclusions regarding the bioaccumulations of sucralose and its breakdown products.*

The FDA did argue that sucralose's low fat solubility, along with animal studies showing limited direct tissue toxicity and no evidence of carcinogenic (cancer-causing) activity in the hydrolysis breakdown products, eliminated any cause for concern.

I disagree with the FDA's conclusion because the vast majority of sucralose safety research was done on rats. Rats only absorb an average of 5 percent, while humans have absorbed as much as 27 percent, and therefore it is not an exact model from which to base conclusions.

Moreover, please remember that the FDA does not require independent testing and analysis of food and drug proposals, and their approval of sucralose was entirely based on the data McNeil provided them. We found many inaccuracies in their presentation of their research data to the public; can we trust their reliability in the data they submitted to the FDA for approval?

FDA FINAL RULING ON BIOACCUMULATION OF SUCRALOSE

The available pharmacokinetics data in the petition do not allow the agency to draw definitive conclusions regarding bioaccumulation of sucralose and its metabolites. However, the available evidence on the physicochemical proper-

---

> ties of sucralose, such as low lipid solubility and high water solubility, is not representative of compounds that manifest a high potential for bio-accumulation. In addition, sucralose is relatively poorly absorbed from the gut in humans in that only 11 to 27 percent of the administered dose is absorbed.
>
> Finally, there is little or no evidence of direct tissue toxicity from sucralose in the mouse, rat, and dog, even when administered at high doses for 1 to 2 years. In a practical sense, the absence of tissue toxicity is more important because even if sucralose had accumulated to some limited degree in these animals, no organ toxicity was demonstrated in any of the long-term studies."

Not everyone agrees with the FDA. According to Dr. James Bowen, bio-chemist and physician:

> In the coming months we can expect to see a river of media hype expounding the virtues of Splenda/sucralose. We should not be fooled again into accepting the safety of a toxic chemical on the blessing of the FDA and saturation advertising. In terms of potential long-term human toxicity we should regard sucralose with its chemical cousin DDT, the insecticide now outlawed because of its horrendous long term toxicities at even minute trace levels in human, avian, and mammalian tissues.[92]

I will end this section on digestion with a few key questions to ponder:

If all sucralose safely passes out of your body intact, as McNeil says, then why have hundreds of people written me letters about the serious symptoms they developed once they start using it?

If it is not stored in your body, unlike every other organochlorine, then why do some people have continued symptoms for months after they stop using it?

What happens to someone if they have a decreased ability to detoxify sucralose from their body due to a poor diet, unhealthy lifestyle or disease condition?

Is Sucralose Safe in Preganacy?

Splenda.com states that "Radiolabel studies show that sucralose is not actively transported across the blood-brain barrier, the placental barrier, or the mammary gland."[93] And it assures pregnant women that "Sucralose can be used safely during pregnancy . . . Studies in animal models showed that sucralose is not actively transported across the placental barrier.[94]

However, according an internal FDA memo discussing the distribution of sucralose in pregnant rats, a study McNeil submitted to the FDA but did not publish:[95]

> Sucralose levels in most tissues followed the same pattern as was found in the plasma, but the *brain, fetal tissues and amniotic fluid* rose over a period of 24 hours and then dropped slowly with plasma levels after 24 hours. On repeated dosing, amniotic fluid should *accumulate* TGS [sucralose] excreted by the fetus . . .[96]

So, on one hand, we have Splenda.com stating that sucralose is safe during pregnancy because the fetus is not exposed to sucralose. On the other hand we have rat studies which clearly show that sucralose does enter the brain, the fetus, the placenta and the amniotic fluid. Not only will the fetus be exposed to the sucralose, but when it excretes the sucralose, it will be bathed in ever increasing levels of sucralose in the amniotic fluid, increasing the possibility of health risks (to both mother and fetus).

Splenda.com also assures nursing mothers that:

> Sucralose can be used safely by nursing mothers . . . Radiolabel studies show that sucralose is not actively transported across . . . the mammary gland.[97]

Nursing mothers read this statement and assume that it is safe to consume sucralose while breast-feeding their baby, because it sounds like sucralose does not contaminate the breast milk. But the same rat study that McNeil submitted to the FDA directly contradicts this, finding:

> The oral administration of sucralose revealed . . . levels of *radioactivity [radioactive sucralose] in maternal milk comparable to the amount appearing in the plasma of female rats.*[98]

Previous studies did not show adverse effects on baby rats who were fed the resulting breast milk. But that's a very different thing from claiming that there was no sucralose in the breast milk at all.

Studies on Pregnant Animals and Their Offspring

A study on four groups of 16–18 pregnant rabbits tested with high doses of sucralose had disturbing results.[99] A total of twelve rabbits in the study died (one in the control group and eleven in the sucralose groups). The experimenters said that only two of these deaths were due to sucralose treatment, and 5–6 died from compliations of the tube feedings.

But there's even more interesting data. Nine rabbits in the high dose sucralose group at 450 times the estimated daily intake (EDI) became pregnant, but four of them *aborted* their fetuses. None of the rabbits in the other groups aborted. There were also decreases in the mean number of viable young per litter and gastrointestinal tract disturbances in this high-dose group. Interestingly, if you only read the abstract of this study, as many people do, you would find the McNeil researchers' conclusion was ". . . maternal consumption of high levels of sucralose during the period of organogenesis has *no effect on normal fetal development* in the rat or rabbit." No effect? Half the fetuses aborted, and they call that "no effect"?

The researchers dismissed the deaths as likely being unique to rabbits, since they did not observe similar reactions in mice, rats, or dogs. They did believe that the deaths were probably related to the higher absorption rate of sucralose in rabbits, which has been mentioned previously. So now you can see the central importance of how much sucralose is absorbed into your body.

The FDA Final Rule discusses this study and noted that rabbits had gastrointestinal disturbance from the sucrolose. However, it concluded that while maternal and fetal toxicity were observed in the rabbit at the high-dose level, there was no evidence of teratogenicity (birth defects), so therefore sucralose is not teratogenic in rabbits. The FDA rule also noted that sucralose did not have maternal or fetal deaths in rats fed up to 1 percent of sucralose in their diet. Amazingly, this is one of the studies used to support the assertion that sucralose is safe in human pregnant women.

There were four pregnant rat studies[100] mentioned in the FDA Final Rule. Three of these studies found significantly retarded growth in both the offspring and the adult rats fed high doses of sucralose, but did not find any other significant effects. Because none of the animal studies showed birth defects, the FDA concluded that sucralose was safe in pregnancy at the ADI (acceptable daily intake) of 5 mg/kg/d.

If sucralose is as safe in pregnancy as they assert, why haven't they ever tested it on pregnant women? Is it perhaps too risky to take the chance? If they were to find adverse risks for human mothers and fetuses, like the severe effects that occurred in the pregnant rabbits who were fed sucralose, it would be devastating for their advertised image of sucralose as a product that is safe and nontoxic for everyone.

Is Sucralose Safe for Your Children?

No one knows if sucralose is safe for children; it has never been tested on children. What we do know, however, is that children's bodies are ill-equipped to handle any kind of toxins; because of their small body weight, they absorb much more toxins by weight than adults do.

Furthermore, a child's immune system is not fully developed until the seventh year, and they are less able to break down certain toxins and excrete them. Molecules of many toxins, such as lead and other metals, are small enough to pass through the placenta to the fetus and can weaken or break down the protective screen of the blood-brain barrier, which can impair brain development. Childhood is a period of critical organ development and fast growth; if there is a disruption in this organ development, it may be irreparable.[101]

Both children and developing fetuses are very sensitive to the effects of organochlorine such as pesticides and sucralose. A National Cancer Institute Study showed that children exposed to pesticides had increased risks of several cancers, and that the rise in rates was greater for children than for adults. A University of Southern California study showed that children were 6.5 times more likely to develop leukemia when their parents used garden pesticides.

A University of North Carolina study showed that mothers who lived within a mile of an agricultural area and were exposed to certain pesticides during weeks three to eight of pregnancy had twice the risk of having a stillbirth. Another study found that babies had a 70-percent increased risk for congenital defects if their mothers used pesticides around the house, or lived within a quarter mile of an agricultural crops, during the month before conception and the first trimester of pregnancy.[102]

There is no need whatsoever to feed your kids Splenda. Please let them decide for themselves if they want to take the risk when they are old enough to read this book but in the meantime, nourish your children with a whole foods diet.

FDA Response To Concerns About Sucralose

1. Genotoxicity Testing

Genototoxcicity is defined as an agent that damages cellular DNA, resulting in mutations or cancer Sucralose and its hydrolysis products showed weakly genotoxic responses in some of the McNeil genotoxicity tests. Furthermore, 1,6-DCF is known to associate with DNA in all tissues which increases the risk for mutagenicity. Several consumer groups asked the FDA for more testing on these issues to prove safety. Despite these findings, the FDA stated:

> . . . as demonstrated in the 2-year rodent bioassays (E053, E055, and E057), there was no evidence of carcinogenic activity for either sucralose or its hydrolysis products. Results from these chronic carcinogenicity studies supersede the results observed in the genotoxicity tests because they are more direct and complete tests of carcinogenic potential.

Since then however, a group of Japanese scientists found that sucralose induced DNA damage in gastrointestinal organs in mice and concluded that "more extensive assessment of food additives [such as sucralose] in current use is warranted."[104]

2. Fertility Studies

In one of the rat studies,[105] sucralose was shown to have a long residual time in the testes. Furthermore, there was another McNeil study that showed brown colored sucralose had a negative effect on sperm (E107)— McNeil claimed that this study was irrelevant because the sucralose they used in the study was "degraded" into its breakdown products.[106] However, McNeil *did not* exclude the possibility that degradation products of sucralose (possibly 6-chlorosugars) may have caused the original antifertility effects. (FDA Final Rule. Federal Register: April 3, 1998 (Vol. 63, Num. 64), available: cfsan.fda.gov/~lrd/fr980403.html and Malkins Legal Firm To: FDA. Letter. September 27, 1999. Re: Sucralose Food Additive Petition).

Other chlorinated monosaccharides, similar to the structure of sucralose, have caused male infertility in rats. McNeil, therefore, submitted four different studies to the FDA to assess the antifertility potential of sucralose in male rats.

The FDA stated that these studies were only fourteen days in duration, and the minimum time needed to cover the cycle of spermatogenesis was seventy days. However, the FDA said that no additional studies were needed, due to a previous reproductive study that lasted ten weeks and showed no infertility in the rats.[107]

3. Chronic Toxicity/Carcinogenicity Studies

The studies done on mice and rats fed sucralose for 52–104[108, 109] weeks and other animal studies have shown the following adverse effects:

- **Reduced growth rate** in newborn and adult rats at levels above 500 mg/kg/d[110]

- **Decreased red blood cells** in mice (sign of anemia) at levels above 1,500 mg/kg/d[111]

- **Shrunken thymus** in rats at 3,000 mg/kg/d[112]

- **Decreased thyroxine levels** (thyroid function) in male rats at 0.3% and 1.0% of the diet.

  According to McNeil, since this only occurred on male rats, and no abnormalities were observed with the thyroid tissue, this was considered insignificant.

- **Mineral losses** (magnesium and phosphorus)

  McNeil stated that these patterns were variable and at times not dose related so they were not significant.

- **Decreased urination**

- **Enlarged colon** in rats at .3% and higher
    The FDA Final Rule states cecal (colon) enlargement is often seen with poorly absorbed substances and is not significant.

- **Enlarged liver and brain** at .3% in female and 3% in male rats
    McNeil stated these were insignificant due to a lack of a dose response.

- **Shrunken ovaries** in rats at 1% and 3%.

- **Enlarged and calcified kidneys** in rats at 3%.
    McNeil stated this is often seen with poorly absorbed substances and was of no toxicological significance. The FDA Final Rule agreed that these findings are common in aged female rats and are not significant.

- **Increased adrenal cortical hemorrhagic degeneration** in rats at 3%.
    McNeil stated that this is a variable finding common in aged rats and not toxicologically significant.

- **Increased cataracts** in male rats at 3%.
    McNeil stated that cataracts were discovered upon microscopic sections of the eye tissue and that this was not as accurate as in-life ophthalmological examinations and did not reveal any treatment-related ocular findings.

- **Abnormal liver cells** in rats at .3%
    The FDA Final Rule states that this was only marginal and probably not treatment related due to the severity of the lesion was not concomitant with the dosage.

McNeil concluded that all of these findings could be explained by reasons other than sucralose toxicity and were insignificant. This seems to be a pattern in all of McNeil's study conclusions. I find it suspect that for every single adverse finding in the animal studies, McNeil always has some rationale that renders it "insignificant." Their downplaying every harmful finding makes it seem as if they are more interested in making sucralose appear safe than making sure that the people are not harmed.

The FDA concluded that most of these findings had no toxicological significance and those that did, such as the decrease in thymus weight and the decreased red blood cells, would not be a problem because they occurred at doses of sucralose much higher than what people would consume.

As a physician, I beg to differ. I believe that these findings are not of "no significance." Many of these are symptoms of serious pathology.

4. Growth Retardation

Numerous studies showed that animals treated with sucralose had significant growth retardation (up to 26 percent) for both adult and newborn rats fed sucralose, and also showed significantly decreased birth weights for newborns. Growth retardation at levels greater than 10 percent are an indication of toxicity.

McNeil countered that the growth retardation had nothing to do with sucralose toxicity, and instead was due to decreased eating because the sucralose-laden food was unpalatable.[113]

But the FDA stated in the final rule that the sucralose was indeed responsible for the growth retardation at a concentration of 3 percent of the diet and therefore it would be safe if people consumed sucralose below that level.

5. Damage to the Immune System

Immunotoxicity is a potentially important issue with sucralose because organochlorides are notorious for causing immune system damage. And indeed, the studies done on rats showed that sucralose affected numerous immunological parameters,[114] such as decreased thymus weights, decreased leukocytes and lymphocytes (white blood cells), and decreased size of the spleen and thymus by as much as 40 percent.[115]

McNeil argued that all of these changes were secondary effects due to palatability-related reduced food intake. To demonstrate this, McNeil conducted feeding tube studies to eliminate the variable of food intake. The results for the mid-dose group were inconclusive, but the very high-dose group (3,000/mg/kg/d) showed that sucralose does significantly decrease the weight of the thymus gland. No other immunological parameters were affected. The FDA Final Rule concluded that the lower doses of 1500 mg/kg was the level at which immunotoxicity was observed.[116]

Acceptable Daily Intake

The animal studies did find that sucralose had a variety of toxic effects at high doses. The FDA took this information and estimated the "no observed effect" for each kind of toxicity, gave it a 100 times safety margin, and came up with an Acceptable Daily Intake (5 mg/kg/bw/d) that they guessed would be safe for humans to consume.[117] The problem is, I've received hundreds of letters from people having toxic reactions to sucralose who were well under the ADI (some were consuming it at miniscule levels of one packet ([11 mg]) a day).[118]

According to Sucralose Toxicity Information Center Website: one reason for this is the wide variation of humans in their ability to detoxify their body from chemicals. One person may not experience noticeable effects until a high dose of 10 mg/kg is reached, while another may experience chronic toxicity effects of 1 mg/kg or less—a variation of 10 times within the human population. It is well known in toxicology that chemicals are much more toxic in humans than they are in rodents or even monkeys. This is why they have a 100-fold safety margin. Moreover, the website states:

> In order to estimate a potential safe dose in humans, one must divide the lowest dose in given to rodents that was seen to have any negative effects on their thymus glands, liver or kidneys by 100. That dose is then known as the maximum Tolerable Daily Intake (TDI) [ADI] for lifetime use. Keep in mind that the TDI is just an estimate. Some chemicals are much more than 10 times more toxic in humans than in rodents (or will cause cancer in humans in low-dose, long-term exposure and do not cause cancer in rodents at all). A person ingesting the TDI for some chemical may find that it causes cancer or immune system or neurological problems after many years or decades of use. So, if the manufacturer claims that the dose was equivalent to 50 diet sodas, then the TDI would be *one half (1/2) of a diet soda, and even that dose may or may not be safe.* (Gold, Mark. Sucralose Toxicity Information Center. Available: holisticmed.com/splenda)

Dr. Ralph Heywood is the Scientific Executive of Huntingdon Life Sciences, one of the largest animal labs in Europe concerned with screening drugs, and he estimated that "The best guess for the correlation of adverse reactions in man and animal toxicity data is somewhere between 5 per cent and 25 per cent." (R. Heywood, "Animal Toxicity Studies: Their Relevance For Man," eds. C. E. Lumley and S. R. Walker [Quay Pub: 1990])

Furthermore, for a 150-pound person, an ADI of 5 mg/kg equals 340 mg of sucralose. Let's say a 150-pound woman bakes cookies using Splenda No Calorie Sweetener or makes fourteen cups of lemonade. Either recipe calls for one-and-a-half cups of Splenda No Calorie Sweetener, which contains 4,125 mg of sucralose—an amount that exceeds her safe intake by at least twelve times (perhaps more, since sucralose breakdown products after baking have not been studied).

To consume sucralose is a unknown risk. What are the long-term effects of sucralose on humans over ten, twenty, or thirty years, and over a lifetime? No one—not McNeil, not the FDA, no one—has any idea. Is saving a few calories worth the risk? Only you can decide.

"Splenda No Calorie Sweetener" Is a Lie

Artificial sweeteners are far sweeter than sugar and 316 times the price, and so Splenda® No Calorie Sweetener, and for that matter all of the powdered artificial sweeteners, are mixed with bulking agents like dextrose, sucrose, and maltodextrin to make the sweeteners more palatable, affordable, and easier to handle and bake with.

What the unsuspecting public doesn't realize though is that the bulking agents are another form of SUGAR.

So just what exactly are dextrose and maltodextrin? Well, you might be familiar with them under their more common names; *dextrose* is another term for glucose. This is the same as refined corn sugar and is the sugar that actually circulates in your blood: it's what is being measured when your blood sugar levels are checked. *Maltodextrin* is the scientific term for corn syrup solids composed primarily of fructose and glucose in a starch form.

I already covered the dangers of high-fructose corn syrup in chapter 1, including the fact that high-fructose corn syrup has played a very significant role in the obesity epidemic. Eating sugars like corn glucose and high-fructose corn syrup will raise your blood sugar. Chronically elevated blood sugars can lead to obesity and diabetes.

All Artificial Sweetener Packets Are at Least 96 Percent Sugar

And Splenda is even WORSE—99 percent of Splenda® No Calorie Sweetener is sugar. It is only 1 percent sucralose.

No one is dropping in pure sucralose into their coffee. They are pouring in packets that are 99 percent pure sugar.

However, despite the fact that Splenda No Calorie Sweetener is 99 percent refined and caloric sugar, the food labeling laws legally allow them to describe their product as being "sugar-free" if the serving size is less than .5 grams of sugar and "calorie-free" if the serving size is less than 5 calories. This is why on a bag of Splenda No Calorie Sweetener you will see that the serving sizes are tiny: .5 grams (1 tsp.) for the granular and 1 gram for the packets. A 1-gram packet contains 4 calories but because this is under the 5 calorie rule, the calories get written off.[119]

SPLENDA NO CALORIE SWEETENER IS A VERY EXPENSIVE SUGAR

Sugar costs $0.35 per pound industrially, or about $0.72 cents at the retail level. Despite the fact that Splenda No Calorie Sweetener is 99 percent sugar, a granulated bag of it costs $16.50 per pound and a box of packets costs $27.52 per pound! Splenda consumers are paying *23–38 times more* for a bag that is 99 percent sugar because the advertising on the Splenda No Calorie Sweetener products claims that it is "sugar-free."

ART'S STORY

Art, a sixty-seven-year-old man, has had type 2 diabetes for many years. He was following strict nutritional guidelines to prevent his diabetes from progressing. His blood sugar was relatively well-managed, and ranged between 90 and 125.

Art's girlfriend, as part of her effort to make healthy choices for his diet, started buying Splenda in the supermarket—it was, after all, advertised as having no calories and no carbohydrates, and being completely safe for diabetics. They began to use it daily in their coffee, tea, and cereal.

Soon after, Art's blood sugar started to go through the roof—regularly going above 200. This went on for several worrisome months. Then one day, when Art and his girlfriend read the ingredients listed on the Splenda box more closely, they were appalled to discover that it actually did have sugar in it, in the form of dextrose and maltodextrin. They immediately removed Splenda from their diet—and Art's blood sugar immediately returned to his normal levels.

More Deception for Diabetics

The research studies have shown that sucralose does not raise blood sugars and therefore is "safe" for diabetics. But there are no research studies to show that the mixture of sucralose and refined and chemically altered corn or starch-based maltodextrin/dextrose sold as Splenda No Calorie Sweetener does not raise blood sugars. I suspect McNeil never studied the effects of the Splenda No Calorie Sweetener because they knew darn well what would happen if they did: blood sugars would increase.

Although normally maltodextrin and dextrose contain just as many calories and carbohydrates as table sugar (1 tsp. contains 15 calories and 4 grams of carbohydrate), there is an aeration method that can be used with the maltodextrin to make it light and fluffy and reduce the calories by 50 percent.

I am assuming McNeil uses the aerated maltodextrin, because the www.Splenda.co.uk Web site states that 1 tsp. of Splenda No Calorie Sweetener contains only 2 calories and 0.5 grams of carbohydrate. Although these calorie and carbohydrate amounts seem small, they *may still have a harmful effect on blood sugars.* Dr. Richard Bernstein, a diabetologist with over twenty-three years experience, in his national bestseller *Dr. Bernstein's Diabetes Solution,* tells all diabetics to avoid powdered artificial sweeteners:

When [artificial sweeteners] are sold in powdered form, under such brand names as Sweet'n Low, Equal, The Sweet One, Sunett, Sugar Twin, Splenda® No Calorie Sweetener and others, these products usually contain a sugar [maltodextrin/dextrose] to increase bulk, and will *rapidly raise blood sugar.*[120]

The carbohydrate count in Splenda® No Calorie Sweetener starts adding up in the larger doses that are required for recipes. One cup of Splenda® No Calorie Sweetener contains 96 calories and 32 grams of carbohydrates and would dangerously and rapidly raise the blood sugars of a diabetic— when all the while he or she thinks that it is calorie-free and sugar-free.

Based solely on the fact that there has never been a human clinical trial on the blended product Splenda® No Calorie Sweetener, which is 99 percent sugar, it would seem prudent for the FDA to instruct McNeil and the other artificial sweetener companies to immediately remove from Splenda's product packaging and marketing materials: "Suitable for people with diabetes" as this is, in my view, false and misleading.

I have never reviewed or been made aware of a study that established Splenda as being safe for people with diabetes.

KATHY'S STORY

Kathy had been trying to lose weight for a long time but resisted drinking diet sodas because she thought that aspartame was poisonous. But when Splenda came on the market, claiming to be made from sugar, she was delighted, thinking that finally a safe no-calorie sweetener was available. She began drinking diet root beer.

Soon, she was experiencing pain in her hips and legs, mainly at night. She could hardly sleep, and if she needed to use the bathroom, she could barely walk.

She wondered if her mattress was causing the problem, so she got a select comfort bed. That did no good, so she tried memory foam, then a latex mattress. The pain continued. Visits to her doctor provided no cure. She began to take painkillers before going to bed.

One day, she decided to stop buying soda because she was tired of dealing with all the cans. To her surprise, the pain in her legs went away, but at first she didn't make the connection. After a while she bought a box of Splenda® No Calorie Sweetener so she could sweeten her own drinks.

The pain in her legs immediately returned. She started to realize that the pain had gone away shortly after she stopped drinking soda, and returned when she added Splenda back into her diet. She immediately stopped using Splenda. After a month, her hips and legs didn't bother her at all.

Reported Side Effects from Sucralose

The Splenda.com Web site states that the conclusion of the safety studies was that there are "No known side effects" and "No toxicity" associated with sucralose use.[121] If there are no side effects, then why have hundreds of people written me letters describing the horrific symptoms they experienced many times after consuming sucralose? The following list contains some of the most common symptoms listed in the sucralose testimonials on Mercola.com. These symptoms have been observed within a twenty-four-hour period following consumption of sucralose products. If you are experiencing any of these symptoms, you may consider stopping your use of products containing sucralose:

- Skin—Redness, itching, swelling, blistering, weeping, crusting, rash, eruptions, or hives (itchy bumps or welts). (Rashes are one of the most common complaints in people who react to sucralose. They are a sign that the immune system has gone haywire in response to a foreign invader.)

- Lungs—Wheezing, tightness, cough, or shortness of breath

- Head—Dry mouth and sinuses; swelling or inflammation of the face, eyelids, lips, tongue, or throat; headaches and migraines

- Nose—Stuffy nose, runny nose, sneezing

- Eyes—Red (bloodshot), itchy, swollen, or watery
- Stomach—Bloating, gas, pain, constipation, nausea, vomiting, diarrhea, or bloody diarrhea
- Heart—Chest pains, palpitations or fluttering
- Joints—Joint pains or aches
- Neurological—Seizures, anxiety, anger, panic, insomnia, dizziness, spaced-out sensation, mood swings, depression
- Other—Bleeding readily without clotting, blood in urine, menstrual delay or missed period, night sweats, numbness of the limbs

Perhaps McNeil states that sucralose does not have side effects because many of these symptoms cannot even be identified in the majority of McNeil's trials, as they were done on animals. When was the last time your dog or cat told you they felt depressed? Has the rabbit in your backyard ever complained to you of migraines?

If you experience any adverse affects as a result of consuming Splenda or any other artificial sweetener, you can find out how to report your symptoms to the FDA at SweetDeception.com/Report.

Although people have been reporting their symptoms from aspartame to the FDA for over a decade, and they have fallen on deaf ears, perhaps this time it will make a difference.

STEVE'S STORY

Steve was trying out the low-carb "Protein Power" diet. He had tried a variety of artificial sweeteners to help assuage his sweet tooth. The first time Splenda® No Calorie Sweetener became available, he ordered it from Canada. The box sported the message "Can be used just like sugar in ANY recipe."

Steve took the box at its word and decided to make caramel. He poured a cup of Splenda® No Calorie Sweetener into the pot and turned the heat on, paying careful attentive to make sure it wouldn't burn as it melted. But the Splenda® No Calorie Sweetener didn't melt; instead, the flakes started browning. Curious to see what it smelled like, Steve stuck his nose over the pan and inhaled.

He immediately fell to the floor in a coughing fit. It felt like battery acid had been poured into his nostrils. In a panic, he called poison control. The burning sensation in his nose persisted for several hours and he had painful dry coughs for days afterward. The caramel was inedible. It tasted like it was full of acid and cayenne pepper.

Deciding that his "do it yourself" approach might have caused the problem, he found a Web site that sold Splenda-sweetened low-carb caramel. He ordered two bags and sampled half a bag when it arrived.

Within an hour, he began to experience intense intestinal cramping and nausea. He felt as if he had "swallowed hot lava." After a period of excruciating agony, the symptoms finally went away.

He never touched Splenda again.

Can You Bake With It?

With the exception of Splenda, no other artificial sweeteners have been approved for baking because their chemical composition changed upon heating, making them unsafe for consumption. Yet again, Splenda is the exception to the rule, as McNeil proudly proclaims on Splenda.com that:

> SPLENDA® No Calorie Sweetener can be used almost anywhere you use sugar in cooking and baking—but its baking properties are different from sugar.

What a boon to civilization. Now we can make low-calorie, sugar-free desserts to our hearts' content and have no guilt, which is why people are willing to pay twenty-three times more for Splenda than the price of table sugar. Splenda's ability to be used in baking certainly is one of the big reasons for its raging success.

However, it is important to note that in studies, sucralose has been shown to break down in hot acidic conditions. Even though not all baking environments are acidic, there is still the problem of dechlorination occurring when sucralose is heated to a high temperature. Drs. Goldsmith and

Grice of McNeil Nutritionals state that sucralose can degrade at a somewhat faster rate when subjected to elevated temperatures for prolonged periods of time.[122] Sucralose is generally stable at 75°F. However, when baking, the oven temperature is usually at least 350°F for 25–60 minutes.

The Material Safety Data Sheet for sucralose states that "if subjected to elevated temperatures, [it] may break down with the release of potentially hazardous decomposition gases including carbon dioxide and hydrogen chloride." Hydrogen chloride is a toxic corrosive gas. Inhalation of the fumes can cause coughing, choking, inflammation of the nose, throat, and upper respiratory tract, and in severe cases it can cause pulmonary edema, circulation system failure, and death. That's why Steve, in the case study mentioned above, experienced such a severe reaction from cooking his Splenda caramel. In my medical opinion he was poisoned with toxic chlorine gas.

But toxic gases aside, how does it compare to table sugar in taste tests? We found two articles[123, 124] on the Internet in which chefs prepared desserts made with sugar and compared them to desserts made with Splenda and had blind taste testers provide their comments.

All of the desserts made with table sugar came out perfect and delicious, and all of the desserts made with Splenda were a bitter disappointment. Both the chefs and the testers preferred the recipes made with natural table sugar hands down. Here are some excerpts from the articles about the desserts made with Splenda:

> For pastry chefs like Falkner, Luchetti and Weil, working with Splenda® was like a trip to an alternate universe where nothing went as it should. They found a pattern with the baked items. The ones made with the sugar rose, had a moist, light texture and browned nicely. The ones made with Splenda® were flat, dense, pale and dry.
>
> The brownies made with Splenda® thudded out of their pan in one thin, dense square. "It looks like a pot holder," cracked Falkner. "Or a floor tile," said Luchetti.
>
> The Splenda® left the ice cream so hard it broke into shards when scooped, and made a custard that Luchetti said "looks like airline scrambled eggs."

Cut-out cookies made with the artificial sweetener were dry, heavy, powdery and distinctly lacking in flavor. One reviewer remarked, "I'd much rather eat an overbrowned one of these [sugar] cookies than any of those ([Splenda® cookies])."

For the chefs, the trade-off in pleasure delivered by a sweet treat isn't worth it. At Citizen Cake's bakery counter, customers sometimes ask Falkner to make them a Splenda cake. She tells them, "I'll make you half a real cake."

Adds Luchetti, "It's like, would you rather have one great glass of wine or four glasses of bad wine?"

One of our consultants, a PhD pharmaceutical and food chemist, had conducted off-the-record exit interviews at the Institute of Food Technology National Expo with six frustrated ex-McNeil employees over a two-year period prior to FDA approval, who consistently said that "sucralose does not work in heated items; the third hydrocarbon link between the three chlorine molecules and sucrose is unstable when heated and gives baked goods a horrible chlorine aftertaste. This fact was ignored by McNeil and Tate & Lyle management for fear of further delay in approval."

Sucralose Also Not Friendly to the Environment

Not only does sucralose have the potential to cause you health problems and ruin your desserts, but it is also harming the planet you live on by contributing to serious pollution problems from the U.S. factories that produce it.

In 1998, after analyzing over thirty studies Tate & Lyle submitted that evaluated the effect of sucralose in water and waste streams, and its potential effects on fish, invertebrates, and other species, the FDA's final ruling on sucralose concluded that sucralose "will not have significant impact on the human environment and an environmental impact statement is not required."

However, eight years later, when we examine the sucralose manufacturing plant, we find something different. According to Scorecard.org, a pollution information site, the sucralose-producing plant in McIntosh, Alabama, ranks in the top 80–90 percentile among the Dirtiest/Worst U.S. facilities for total environmental releases. This is no small feat when you consider many of the steel, coal, plastics, and pesticide industries that exist in our country. In 2002, McNeil Nutritionals' sucralose factory produced *9.5 million pounds* of total production waste, of which *200,000 pounds were released into the air and water.*[125]

According to records on file with the Environmental Protection Agency's Toxic Release Inventory (TRI) database, the following chemicals were released from the McIntosh, Alabama plant:

- Cyclohexane—processing aid
- Dimethylamine—Manufacture; byproduct; process chemical as impurity

> Dimethylamine is a suspected cardiovascular/blood and gastrointestinal/liver toxicant, immunotoxicant, neurotoxicant, respiratory toxicant, and skin and sense organ toxicant. It is ranked as one of the most hazardous compounds (worst 10 percent) to ecosystems and human health.

- N,N-Dimethylformamide—Reactant; processing aid
- Nitrate Compounds—Byproduct
- Phosgene—Byproduct and reactant
- Chlorine—Reactant

Other chemicals released into the air and water include: 3,3'Dichlorobenzidine, dihydrochloride, creosotes, dimethyl sulfate, N-Methylolacrylamide, N-Nitrosomethylvinylamine, propachlor,acetaldehyde, 2-Nitropropane, and 1,4-Dichloro-2-Butene.

This data is from 2002. The supply of sucralose has increased considerably since then, so it would seem reasonable to assume that the amount of chemicals released into the environment has also increased considerably.

Recently, twenty-nine residents living near the sucralose plant are filing a class action lawsuit against Tate & Lyle because the plant has decreased property values from the noise and air pollution, and many have experienced medical problems with symptoms similar to phosgene gas exposure.[126]

Phosgene and chlorine gas were used as poison gas warfare agents in

World War I. There were responsible for the hospitalization or death of almost 1,400,000 soldiers.

Hundreds of residents have gathered to protest Tate & Lyles plans to double the capacity of the plant in 2006. "There's gonna be a lot more fresh graves," one middle-aged woman said, recalling how many neighbors had been buried because of what she described as lung problems.[127]

In 2002, the following Pollutants were released from the McNeil sucralose plant in McIntosh, AL:

	AIR RELEASES	WATER RELEASES
	(IN POUNDS)	
Suspected Cardiovascular/ BloodToxicants	1,702	167,530
Suspected Developmental Toxicants	11,533	5,892
Suspected Immunotoxicants	1,702	
Suspected Kidney Toxicants	11,533	5,982
Suspected Gastrointestinal/ Liver Toxicants	13,235	5,892
Suspected Neurotoxicants	16,713	5,892
Suspected Reproductive Toxicants	11,533	5,892
Suspected Respiratory Toxicants	13,235	5,892
Suspected Skin or Sense Organ Toxicants	13,235	5,892

All data was obtained from the EPA's Toxic Release Inventory.
NOTE: Some chemicals are associated with more than one health effect, so their releases may be counted more than one time in this table.

Currently, the plant in McIntosh, Alabama is the sole producer of sucralose. During 2006, the plant is supposed to double production to meet the need for increased demand. Recently, Tate & Lyle announced additional plans to expand production capacity at some of their other plants in order to more than triple sucralose production. The company also intends to finish construction of a new $175 million sucralose plant in Singapore by 2007.[128]

Considering the alarming rate at which Splenda consumption is growing, the impact on our health and the environment is a huge concern.

The Bottom Line: Avoid the Deception

Many people have been deceived into believing that everything the FDA says is safe is indeed truly safe. I hope the evidence I provide in this book will help you to understand that this is merely wishful thinking. It is my hope that you will begin to question the authority of the FDA, and do some research when you consider using any item they have approved that you intend on using for long periods of time.

The FDA has failed to protect you on many occasions. You'll find out in the next two chapters how they failed miserably with Vioxx®, for example.

> According to pharmaceutical chemist Shane Ellison: "To use an organochlorine to make a sweetener defies logic. It is the first organochlorine ever used for human consumption. I would no sooner eat Splenda® than I would eat DDT."

And please remember that drugs have a far more stringent approval process than food additives like Splenda.

What you are faced with is an issue of deceptive advertising. As Michael Jacobson, the executive director of the Center for Science in the Public Interest, states, "'Made from sugar' certainly sounds better than, say, 'Made from chlorinated hydrocarbons,' 'Made in a laboratory,' or 'Fresh from the factory!'"[129]

McNeil Nutritionals is providing the same misleading information in their print and Web-based marketing materials to physicians, who then go on to misinform the general public. Splenda.com encourages physicians to help patients improve their health by eating Splenda instead of sugar. But wouldn't it make more sense to encourage people to make better choices about eating whole, REAL foods?

As an educated consumer, you simply cannot take everything you are told at face value—not from manufacturers, not from the FDA, and not even from physicians. Ask questions. The more answers you know, the more empowered you will be to make the right choice for you.

CHAPTER FIVE:
SWEET FOOD

THE POLITICS OF FOOD

The anti-inflammatory drug Vioxx hit the American market in 1999 and was an instant success. With over twenty million Vioxx users, worldwide sales for Vioxx reached $2.5 billion just four years after it was released.

Since 1999, it is estimated that Vioxx has caused 140,000 heart attacks and killed 60,000 people in the United States alone.[1] The system that was originally designed to protect the public from unsafe drugs had failed miserably.

But it didn't just fail in this one isolated instance. Other deadly drugs that were eventually pulled from the market include Rezulin, Redux, Propulsid, Raxar, Posicor, Lotronex, Duract . . . the list goes on and on.

Something has gone horribly wrong.

Warnings about Vioxx had surfaced long before the dangers became common knowledge. In my free health newsletter on Mercola.com in 1999, before the drug was approved, I documented that there was a report in the *Proceedings of the National Academy of Sciences* that suggested an increased risk of cardiac deaths associated with the drug.[2] I advised my readers to avoid Vioxx and predicted that it would be eventually removed from the market, which it was more than five years later. To my knowledge that was the first public warning of the potential dangers of Vioxx.[3]

But if there were reports that showed the drug was dangerous even before it was FDA approved, how did it manage to get onto the market? Why didn't the FDA stop it? Why didn't the manufacturers hold it back for further safety tests? And why is it that this kind of disaster has happened so many times in recent years? What safety net is in place to stop another drug, food additive, or artificial sweetener from becoming the next Vioxx?

The fact is, our only safety net is full of holes. Manufacturers, concerned more with profit than public safety, now have more say in the process that gets products on the market than the scientists who work at the FDA who evaluate the drug safety. We'll return to the Vioxx story later in the book, in the course of examining the dangerous entanglements between private industry and the FDA.

Truth, Lies, and Conflicts of Interest

The vast majority of citizens of industrialized nations are exposed to artificial sweeteners, knowingly or not. Artificial sweeteners are added to a wide variety of foods, drinks, drugs, and hygiene products that are globally consumed. If artificial sweeteners are associated with any potential health hazards whatsoever, this means we are risking the health of nearly the entire population.

So just who is telling you that artificial sweeteners are safe? In essence, the health of our entire population is being entrusted to two main parties: the sleeping watchdogs at the FDA and the very manufacturers of the artificial sweeteners themselves.

The Food Industry—An Empire of Deception

The manufacturers of artificial sweeteners are part of the food industry— a surprisingly small number of international corporations that have taken a tight grip on every aspect of the food production system. These corporations have converted large numbers of small, local suppliers into enormous factory-based systems that radically reduce the health value of food. Lucrative relationships between the largest manufacturers and the largest retailers make it progressively more difficult for smaller food producers to survive. And as large food manufacturers continue to grow in size and power, it becomes even more challenging to find food lacking chemical additives and preservatives.

These businesses exert an enormous amount of influence on the kind of food that is available for your consumption. And the American food supply, under their control, has changed drastically over the past fifty years.

Food no longer comes from local farmers who have developed their techniques through generations of experience. Large machinery, genetic manipulation, pesticides, and herbicides have replaced these time-tested techniques. And most farms no longer bear any resemblance to the happy children's book barnyard scenes in which animals roam freely. Instead, chickens are crammed into cages so tightly that they can barely move. This usually drives them to psychotic types of behavior, so their beaks and claws are cut off to prevent them from killing each other. Cattle are jammed into factory feedlots and are dehorned for similar reasons. Most are kept alive by a lifetime diet of chemicals and antibiotics designed to maximize their growth. They feed on sawdust mixed with ammonia, processed sewage, cardboard scraps, and similar delicacies during their feedlot "fattening" phase.[4]

The American food supply is produced on a massive scale and typically shipped thousands of miles to reach you. Highly processed and refined foods have replaced the fresh, nutrient-dense foods your grandparents enjoyed. Americans have also begun to abandon the practice of cooking at home from scratch, preferring instead to purchase their convenience foods prepared from highly processed packages or from restaurants. Changes in eating habits and food production have led to the almost inescapable presence of additives and preservatives in your food supply. Sadly, the addition of a wide array of chemicals to food is now considered a standard and necessary practice to provide maximum flavor and the lowest possible cost, and food quality is rarely given any serious consideration.

Grocery-store shelves are overrun with nutritionally depleted foods that are destroying your health. Refined foods are stripped of naturally occurring oils, fiber, vitamins, minerals, and other micro-nutrients during the manufacturing process. Tons of chemical compounds are added to the food supply to preserve freshness, alter consistency, enhance flavor, and reduce calories.

Organic, nongenetically modified, nonirradiated, locally produced food, which was once the standard for all Americans, is now considered an unusual alternative that can be found only in a few specialty stores located primarily in large, affluent urban areas. The food industry has shifted away from producing food that your body needs and moved toward producing food products that can generate maximum revenues for their parent corporation.

Who Are the Food Giants?

The poultry industry is one example of how rapidly food production has been transformed. As little as fifty years ago, most farmers raised chickens in small flocks. Many small farms across the nation directly supplied the stores and restaurants that were regionally accessible to them. Today, the majority of chickens are produced from factory farms that work under contracts with just a handful of corporations. Local independent chicken farmers can no longer compete with the price that can be offered by multinational corporations and are slowly being forced to close.

The same change has occurred in the beef industry. In the 1970s, the top four U.S. beef packers controlled 25 percent of the American market. Today, four processing firms control over 80 percent of beef processing through contracts. Meanwhile, twenty feedlots supply food for half of the cattle in the United States.

Every tier of the American food chain is transitioning toward this kind of international corporate control. The most alarming trend is the merging of the agriculture and livestock industries with the chemical and biotechnology industries. In 1980, twenty different corporations supplied 90 percent of agricultural chemicals worldwide. Just ten years later, less than ten companies controlled the sales of agricultural chemicals.

Wal-Mart's Low Prices Worsen the Problem

Global dominance of the food supply by a handful of industrial interests is reinforced by a similar trend toward corporate concentration on the retail side. Corporations like Wal-Mart have openly declared their ambitions toward global dominance.[5]

Originally, Wal-Mart focused on nonconsumable goods; now, their strategy of creating a one-stop superstore that supplies all needs has fueled the addition of groceries to their shelves.

Food on Wal-Mart's shelves must withstand storage and shipment to thousands of retail outlets worldwide; perishable food must have the stereo-typical perfect look as it sits on the store shelves; and it must be bought at the lowest possible prices to ensure the maximum possible profit. The only way to achieve these ends is by purchasing primarily from suppliers that mass-produce highly processed and chemically treated food. The end result of the marriage between large national food producers and retailers is that the choices for tens of millions of consumers are being reduced to only what is offered by a handful of sources.

Retailers the size of Wal-Mart have incredible power over their suppliers. Wal-Mart demands wholesale prices that are almost impossible to meet. Food manufacturers must appease Wal-Mart's demands, or they risk losing the privilege of having their product available at the most important retailer in America. Suppliers are forced to cut corners to lower costs, and it is often at the expense of compromising food quality.[6]

A walk down the aisle of Wal-Mart's food and produce section is an alarming look at the future of the American food supply: The majority of food is processed or preprepared. The vegetables are individually shrink-wrapped in plastic. And the single most ominous aspect is the overwhelming percentage of junk-food options.

Some experts believe that what you see on the shelves at Wal-Mart is a good representation of the current Standard American Diet (SAD).

Of course, very few consumers shop for groceries exclusively at Wal-Mart . . . right now. But the groceries other stores carry are looking increasingly like those of Wal-Mart as they struggle to match prices and find suppliers. There may still be a vast array of breakfast cereals and sodas to choose from, but how much of a choice is it when they are all sweetened, processed, and laden with chemical additives?

Recently Wal-Mart has decided to transition into organic foods, and it is projected that they will be the largest seller of organic foods in the United States.[7] It is a strategy to bring in the "conscientious consumer," which is a growing consumer group. But like everything else at Wal-Mart, the organic food will probably come from countries like China and Mexico where it can be produced cheaply at slave wages[8] and may just put the American organic farmers out of business. This is one of many reasons why I urge my Mercola.com readers to buy produce from their small local farmers as much as possible.

Only the largest of food corporations can meet Wal-Mart's demand for rock-bottom pricing and massive supply needs. You'll find familiar names in those aisles like Coca-Cola, Gerber, Nestle, Monsanto, Proctor and Gamble, Kraft, Quaker, Johnson & Johnson, Pepsi, Kellogg, Heinz, and Mars. But what most people do not realize is that there are even bigger corporate monopolies controlling most of these brands.

Merging Corporations into Multinational Giants

Fierce competition in the food industry forces smaller companies to merge with larger ones. For example, the cigarette giant Philip Morris owns several other brands, including Kraft Foods, Jell-O Desserts, Miller Brewing Company, and Altoid Mints. PepsiCo owns Pepsi, Lay's Potato Chips, and Tropicana Fruit Juice. Nestle owns Carnation Foods, Lean Cuisine, and Butterfinger Candy. There are even more elusive multinational corporate food giants that are rarely in the public spotlight such as ConAgra, Unilever, and Cargill. All of them own a large piece of the food industry pie.

The trend toward multinational corporate control of the food supply has changed the landscape of America. There are a million fewer farms now than there were forty years ago. The average size of a farm has increased by 40 percent, while the productivity of the farm has increased by 80 percent. And the changes in the American food supply have run parallel to the increased prevalence of chronic diseases and obesity.

The details of the growing dominance of every aspect of the food industry by fewer and fewer international corporations could fill the pages of this entire book. And the consolidation and globalization of food manufacturing and retail industry can be expected to continue. It would not be surprising to see, in the near future, only half a dozen large retail organizations dominating the worldwide marketplace, working closely with the dozen or so corporations that are responsible for global food production. Intertwined delicately into this mix would be a few chemical and biotechnology corporations, offering products that artificially support a food industry that is out of balance with what nature can sustain.

Your Poisonous Diet

In developed countries, modern technology has created an abundant food supply that is no longer dependent on geography or season. In the United States, there is enough food to meet the requirements of a population twice its size. Yet, despite our abundance of cheap and plentiful food, the majority of people die from chronic degenerative diseases that are a result of poor diet and lifestyle choices.[9]

The food industry has been incredibly successful at influencing what you eat. The epidemic of obesity, diabetes, and cancer is a testimony to the food industry's success at encouraging you to eat more of the high-calorie junk foods that skyrocket their profits. One of the easiest techniques to sell food is to prey on your addictions. Convenience and sugar are our society's current primary dietary weaknesses.

The prevalence of the overconsumption of junk food has resulted in the increasing appearance of diseases that were previously rarely seen. "Metabolic syndrome," or "syndrome X," is a diagnosis that was developed to account for the millions of people who are overweight, borderline diabetic, and have heart disease.

At the same time, the nearly inescapable chemical additives are dangerously altering the diet of industrialized nations. Humans evolved for thousands of years on the micro- and macronutrients available from plant and animal food. You are genetically programmed to grow and thrive on a naturally derived diet. Nearly all of the chemical compounds added to food have never previously existed on this planet prior to their creation in some chemist's lab. The impact on your health of thousands of food additives, combined with genetically modified and irradiated food, is unstudied and unknown. The majority of the human race is currently engaged in a massive involuntary experiment on a scale that has never been seen in the history of the world.

We are already experiencing some of the results of this experiment in the epidemic of obesity, diabetes, and Alzheimer's that has hit America:

- Two out of three Americans are overweight or obese.

- In 2005, cancer surpassed heart disease as the number one cause of death in Americans under eighty-five.[10]

- Over seventy-three million Americans now have diabetes or pre-diabetes, and it is increasing in epidemic rates.[11]

Projections for Alzheimer's disease are skyrocketing, and it is expected that more then ten million people in the United States will be affected in the next twenty years.[12]

The "Natural Health" Bandwagon

Many health-conscious people believe they can improve their quality of life by eating fresh and seasonal organic produce, drinking clean water, and minimizing their exposure to the multitude of environmental toxins found in our modern world. The steady growth of the market for organic foods, nontoxic cleaning supplies, and natural medicine is evidence that a natural lifestyle has become increasingly popular.

The multinational corporations of the food industry are not happy with this cultural shift—especially since they are not simply the companies using pesticides on their farms; they are also generally the companies selling them. Large international businesses generally have their fingers in many pies, and the same firms that bring you processed and genetically modified foods are often also the ones bringing you pesticides, herbicides, fertilizer, pharmaceutical drugs, preservatives, and food additives such as artificial sweeteners. For example, the multinational corporation Monsanto has produced saccharine, pharmaceuticals, aspartame, GMO seeds, herbicides, and pesticides.[13]

Johnson & Johnson is another example. They produce artificial foods, such as Splenda and Benecol® spread (butter substitute), and a large range of health-care products from allergy drugs to wound care.[14]

It's clearly in these companies' best interest to convince you that their new chemical compounds represent important and necessary developments in food manufacturing, improvements in farming, and advancements in medicine. But they are encountering a progressively resistant and growing segment of society that believes that these new chemicals are not only unnecessary but are also threatening genetic balance, damaging the environment, harming their bodies, and perhaps even threatening the very existence of the human species as we now know it.

In my opinion, the companies are attempting to use this to their advantage by misleading you into believing that their synthetic and artificial products are virtually identical to the natural ones, spinning half-truths like advertising a synthetic chlorinated hydrocarbon like Splenda is "made from sugar so it tastes like sugar." The companies don't even want to allow labels on food like "organic" or "genetically modified;"[15] they know that informed consumers might avoid their products.

The food industry has developed a dependence on selling cheap, nutrient-depleted, processed junk food in order to increase or maintain their profits. Americans are reaping the results of this experiment and have become overweight and chronically ill from their reliance on the food industry's tempting offerings. Zero-calorie sweeteners and zero-cholesterol oils are designed to keep you gorging on chips, candy, and soda with the perception that you are improving your diet. So they create "foods" like artificial sweeteners or the notorious Olestra.

Olestra, used as a low-calorie fat substitute in potato chips, can, at the very least, cause an embarrassing and messy leaky anus—but it can also lead to cramps, diarrhea, bleeding, or incontinence. This is the kind of chemical that is being promoted as a healthier substitute for real food.

What Is Wrong with This Picture?

Even so, the initial concept of artificial sweeteners sounds innocent enough—develop and market a sweetener three hundred to ten thousand times sweeter than sugar, with zero calories. As obesity and diabetes rates rise to epidemic proportions, a successful zero-calorie sweetener could save the world from its addiction to sweet foods. People can remain addicted to, and continue to consume, soda, candy, cookies, and cakes to their heart's content without any consequences. They can keep their normal body weight and avoid developing heart disease or diabetes.

So what is going wrong?

The problem is that enormous amounts of money are lost if a manufacturer admits that such a product is actually unsafe. It requires millions of dollars to develop, patent, and market these products, and manufacturers stand to make billions if their product is successful. If you hold the patent on an artificial sweetener with a similar taste and texture to that of regular sugar, your profit potential is extraordinary. The market for these calorie-reduced diet products, already in the billions of dollars, continues to grow at an astounding, near-exponential pace.

In spring 2005, Pepsi-Cola North America announced its plans to add Splenda to a newly reformulated Pepsi ONE. Their marketing pitch was a new full-flavored cola taste with only one calorie. Sugar addicts who had avoided the bitter aftertaste of the older artificial sweeteners could now switch over to Pepsi ONE without compromising flavor or worrying about their waistline.

This is where the initial innocent idea of an artificial sweetener gets a life of its own. Pepsi spent millions marketing Pepsi ONE, which is essentially comarketing for Splenda. Now we have two multinational corporations with more interest in their bottom-line profit than in any data that might shed light on the potential health hazards of these artificial sweeteners. And, in the case of a chemical like sucralose that had never before been used by humans, this creates a situation that could be hazardous to the health of hundreds of millions or even billions.

It's easy to understand why it is necessary to question the opinions of the manufacturers of artificial sweeteners. When you buy a house, do you trust the current owner to tell you the truth about its condition? Absolutely not! A real-estate agent, an inspector, and an assessor are available to help you make an informed and wise decision.

The food industry does everything in its power to convince you that the products they are selling you are healthy, whether or not they truly are. They employ marketing geniuses that are experts at using public-relations campaigns designed to convince you that a healthy lifestyle consists of using chemicals that taste sweet but are (according to them, at least) not actually absorbed. They use the manipulation of government regulatory agencies, the media, and scientific literature to promote the concept that using artificial chemicals can result in better nutrition.

After reading this chapter, you will be able to better identify techniques the marketing geniuses use to manipulate your opinion. This is intended to help you make informed decisions as you consider the onslaught of information aimed at convincing you that highly processed and artificial foods are healthy—or at least do no harm.

The Politics of Food

As food-producing and retailing corporations gain global power, they also gain influence. Food companies invest massive resources into creating and protecting an environment conducive to selling their products. Enormous financial and human resources are used to lobby Congress and federal agencies to create policies that favor industry profits. Congress is lobbied for favorable laws, the White House is lobbied for beneficial trade agreements, and the FDA is lobbied for lenient regulations and a user-friendly approval process.

At the same time, behind-the-scenes alliances between food manufacturers and professional nutritional organizations are used to create the illusion of independent expert support. The food industry funds research on food and health that shapes what the public thinks about nutrition. Food corporations also develop relationships with the media to hype select research studies favorable to their agenda. Scientific journals and conferences are funded by food-industry dollars, yet they are still viewed by many as an objective medium to discuss nutrition and health.

These corporations are masters of manipulating public perception of their products. Public-relations firms use scientifically proven techniques to influence your thoughts and feelings surrounding food, nutrition, and diet. The goal of these efforts is to create a population that will consume their products regardless of any potential adverse health effects.

Food and food service companies spend more than $33 billion annually on direct media advertising in magazines, newspapers, radio, TV, and billboards. Most of this enormous sum is used to promote the most highly processed foods. Nearly 70 percent of food advertising is for highly processed convenience foods, candy and snacks, alcoholic beverages, soft drinks, and desserts, whereas just 2.2 percent is for fruits, vegetables, grains, or beans. In 1999, McDonald's spent $627 million, Burger King $404 million, Taco Bell $206 million, and Coca-Cola $174 million on direct media advertising.[16]

Not everyone would label the influence of the food industry over political, academic, and public arenas as a problem. Some would argue that food-industry lobbying is a part of the healthy capitalism that promotes the sale and production of food, which is absolutely necessary to reap all the benefits of the American economy. This argument rapidly breaks down though, because the products being heavily promoted to you as being healthy are actually highly processed, pernicious junk foods that can devastate your health in the same way that smoking tobacco will. You are simply being manipulated into believing that these products are actually healthy.

In the next few decades, when the cost of caring for the victims of heavily marketed junk foods becomes unmanageable, regulatory agencies and policy makers will be forced to intervene. It has been predicted that lawmakers will be prosecuting those corporations that shamelessly promote junk food (especially to children), much like cigarette manufacturers are being prosecuted today. In the future, we may see limits on advertising highly processed convenience foods loaded with sugar, or warnings on synthetic or genetically modified ingredients with unknown effects on human health. But currently you are not protected.

Playing Hardball

Food companies often use hardball strategies to protect their sales, including suing anyone who suggests that their products might have harmful health, safety, or environmental effects. In the late 1980s, for example, a small activist group passed out leaflets to people describing how McDonald's destroys rain forests in order to raise cattle, and why the meat, filled with antibiotics, hormones, and pesticides, was not healthy for people. In response, McDonald's spent $15 million in legal fees to sue two of the group members for libel.[17]

Another famous case involved Oprah Winfrey's on-air comment that she would never eat another burger, in response to her guest's statement that diseased cows are ground up and fed to other cows. The Texas cattle ranchers instituted a $10.3 million class-action suit against Oprah for scaring consumers about eating beef.

Although Oprah eventually won the suit, she had to spend more than $1 million in legal fees to do so.[18] The cattlemen had accomplished their mission; anyone who publicly speaks against food producers faces the potential of an expensive lawsuit to defend against that could have devastating financial consequences, especially in light of the new bankruptcy laws recently enacted in the United States.

Drugs That Earn Profits, but May Kill You in the Process

There have been frequent cases of corporations simply covering up and denying the demonstrably deadly effects of their products. Johnson & Johnson is a New Jersey-based pharmaceutical and toiletries behemoth that, as you'll recall, is the company that distributes Splenda in the United States. Stephen Fried describes their dedication to profit over safety in his book *Bitter Pills*.

Fried's wife may be a real-life victim of one of Johnson & Johnson's controversial antibiotics, Floxin. Floxin is one of ten other quinolone antibiotics that had a questionable safety record. Omniflox, a close relative to Floxin, had just been pulled from the market five months before Fried's wife began taking Floxin.

According to Fried, the pill was initially prescribed to her for a minor infection, but the prescription itself caused her to have a seizure, triggered a debilitating manic-depressive illness, and resulted in *permanent neurological damage*. Floxin is known to stimulate the central nervous system and can cause tremors, restlessness, agitation, nervousness, anxiety, lightheadedness, confusion, hallucinations, paranoia, depression, nightmares, insomnia, and suicidal thoughts or acts. These reactions can occur even with only one dose of the drug.[19]

One example Fried brings up in his book is the story of the diabetes drug Rezulin, which was successfully marketed to millions. Fried explained that, instead of helping diabetic patients, it caused at least 391 documented deaths and hundreds of cases of liver damage before it was finally determined to be unsafe and was withdrawn from the market.

According to Fried, researchers from Warner-Lambert, the manufacturers of Rezulin, knew as early as 1993 of the possibility of life-threatening liver damage from their drug; however, during the approval process, Warner-Lambert lied to the FDA and said that the drug was completely safe and associated with minimal risk, even though they knew of at least twelve patients who had suffered serious cases of liver damage during clinical trials. The FDA approved Rezulin in January 1997.[20]

Almost immediately, Rezulin began causing serious health problems in patients who took it. Despite a rising death toll, Warner-Lambert continued to aggressively market Rezulin to doctors. Rezulin was bringing in $2 million per day in sales, totaling $2.1 billion for Warner-Lambert before the drug was recalled in March 2000. But for over two years before that happened, Warner-Lambert successfully fought off FDA attempts to ban Rezulin. FDA insider, David Graham, testified before congress that the continued marketing of Rezulin during this period probably led to thousands of Americans being severely injured or killed by the drug.[21] Rezulin was finally yanked from the market when the threat of massive class-action lawsuits and potential criminal charges began to outweigh the potential for profit.[22]

IF THE AUTO INDUSTRY OPERATED LIKE BIG PHARMA: FIFTEEN THINGS YOU MIGHT NOTICE

(excerpted from the article by Mike Adams, The Health Ranger at www.newstarget.com[23])

1. Your average car would cost $4.5 million, representing a 30,000 percent markup over cost.

2. That exact same car could be purchased in Mexico or Canada for under $5,000.

3. Automakers would lobby Congress to outlaw or regulate alternative forms of transportation such as bicycles and airplanes.

4. Cars with no safety systems (no seatbelts, no airbags, no crumple zones) would be declared perfectly safe by federal regulators. Car companies, rather than address this lack of safety features, would focus on publicizing the dangers of riding bicycles.

5. The manufacturers of those cars with no safety systems would grow tired of being sued by customers who were injured in their cars, and they would lobby Congress to pass "legal reform" that would immunize all car companies against class-action lawsuits.

---

6. All auto imports would be banned, forcing consumers to buy only U.S. manufactured cars. And if you bought a Toyota and drove it to the United States, you might be arrested or searched.

7. Car companies would heavily publicize the release of new car models each year, but the new models would be "me-too" cars with no real improvements over those made in the 1970s.

8. Car crash dummy tests that produced fatalities and other disturbing data would be censored by the auto industry, never to see the light of day. Any safety scientist who produced such results would be black-balled from ever conducting crash tests again.

9. Car dealers would be visited by hoards of automobile sales reps promising bribes, first-class vacations, free food, and free cars, as long as those car dealers would push the right products on to consumers.

10. Driver's education programs would be cancelled nationwide. Instead of teaching people how to avoid accidents or repair damaged cars, automakers would encourage people to keep buying new cars.

11. Companies would make up new reasons why you need more automobiles, hoping to convince you to buy a dozen or more.

12. Car advertising would show happy, healthy people driving down country highways with the wind blowing through their hair. But once you get the car, you find out it breaks all the time, it doesn't perform as promised, and after a couple of years, it won't even start anymore.

13. Federally mandated warnings about car safety problems would be printed in 6-point type on a tiny label hidden under the driver's seat.

14. Driving certain cars would have unexpected side effects. Driving one car would make you extremely aggressive and violent. Driving another car might make all your muscles hurt. And a third car might make you feel an instant loss of sexual drive.

15. Cars would be sold to you with high-priced features like a sunroof, air conditioning, 6-CD changer, navigation system, and other items, but upon delivery, you would find none of the features you paid for.

When such companies assure you that their other new chemical products are perfectly safe, there is very little historical evidence to support believing their self-serving claims.

Current law does little to stop this kind of corporate malfeasance. When Warner-Lambert was found guilty of fraudulent claims about another product of theirs, Neurontin, they were fined $430 million.[24] But sales for Neurontin are around $2.5 billion per year. The monetary benefit of breaking the rules far outweighs the risk of a comparatively small fine with no jail time.

Making Profits at the Expense of Innocent Babies

In fact, companies place bottom-line profit over the safety of their customers on a fairly routine basis.

Multinational corporations that sell infant formula, like Nestle and Wyeth (American Home Products), make millions of dollars each year by convincing third-world mothers that their formulas are better than breast milk, even though it is a fact that breast milk is vastly superior to any other food for infants. One of the many marketing strategies infant formula manufacturers use is to ingratiate their company with physicians and hospitals with payoffs in cash, gifts, and escort services, in order to get the hospital staff to recommend their infant formulas over breast-feeding.[25]

As a result of using the synthetic formulas, many babies become ill because they are mixed with unsafe drinking water. At the same time, the mothers may run out of money for the formula, but when they attempt to go back to breast-feeding, they cannot because their breast milk has dried up.

At this point, mothers will try to stretch the formula a bit further by adding more water, or going without food themselves so they can afford to continue buying the formula. But this only results in their babies becoming weaker, and most contract diseases as a result of malnutrition that weakens their immune system and makes them susceptible to many infectious diseases. The risk of *death from diarrhea* in the less-developed third-world nations is *twenty-five times higher* for children who are bottle-fed than for those who are breast-fed.[26] *More than one and a half million babies die every year from the cycle of infection and malnutrition associated with infant formulas.*[27]

Monsanto—From Saccharin and Aspartame to Roundup® and Genetic Engineering

Monsanto is a name that you've already heard a few times—the company that was formed to distribute saccharin and was also the manufacturer of aspartame for many years. Recently they have become notorious for their sales practices with Roundup, their best-selling herbicide.[28, 29]

Monsanto uses its market dominance to force farmers to buy both Roundup and expensive, genetically engineered seeds—also produced by Monsanto—which are resistant to the chemical. (Interestingly, during the nineties, Roundup and NutraSweet were being manufactured in the same South American factory. It should be noted that a frequent reason for manufacturing chemicals outside the United States is that the factory regulations are less stringent.)

There are many other examples of their record. Organic Consumers Association, a nonprofit public interest organization focusing on food safety and environmental sustainability, put it as follows: "If you're talking about PCBs, Agent Orange, Bovine Growth Hormone, water privatization, biopiracy, untested/unlabeled genetically engineered organisms, or persecuting small family farmers, you're talking about the Monsanto Corporation."[30]

So how does Monsanto respond when its products are shown to be hazardous? With denials and apparent cover-ups. One jaw-droppingly brazen example of this is their attitude toward Agent Orange—the chlorocarbon they manufactured that was used as a defoliant in the Vietnam War. The dioxin in Agent Orange has been shown to be responsible for kidney and liver damage, cancer, and birth defects, including babies being born without eyes or arms, or missing internal organs. Over the years, numerous lawsuits have been brought against Monsanto as a result, by both American soldiers and Vietnamese citizens.

Their response?

That Agent Orange wasn't responsible at all; in fact, it was *harmless* to humans. They made this amazing claim for decades, supporting their position with a technique that should be familiar to you from chapter 3 on aspartame: error-ridden, self-serving safety studies that they performed themselves.

The scientists at the EPA did not look upon Monsanto's position fondly when they reviewed their claims. EPA researcher Cate Jenkins, PhD, wrote that Monsanto's submitted safety studies on their product revealed "a long pattern of fraud. . . . Monsanto has in fact submitted false information to [the] EPA."[31] She goes on to document that safety studies were riddled with flaws and outright falsifications. Meanwhile, she noted, "available internal Monsanto correspondence in the 1960s shows a knowledge . . . that the dioxin contaminant [of Agent Orange] was responsible for kidney and liver damage."[32]

Somehow, this doesn't inspire a sense of confidence regarding their assurances of the safety of NutraSweet.

Corporations Manipulate Scientific Data

The public relies on properly performed scientific studies to determine health advice. For many consumers and professionals, the randomized, placebo-controlled scientific study represents the pinnacle of scientific truth. Experiments are required to adhere to a specific methodology in order to achieve this level of credibility. In theory, research studies are designed to gather quantitative data that is reproducible and verifiable. An essential part of this equation is that the researchers conducting the experiment are objective and impartial. If a researcher for any reason is biased with an ulterior motive or some underlying conflict of interest, the entire model is invalidated and the results of the experiment cannot be trusted.

The FDA and the public rely on scientists and the scientific method to investigate these newly developed chemicals that are used as food additives, preservatives, and drugs. Food manufacturers are held responsible for conducting research studies with these chemical compounds to prove they do not harm your health.

Unfortunately, by placing the burden of proof in the hands of the same parties that aim to profit, we have lost any semblance of unbiased objectivity, and the validity of the model is hopelessly inaccurate.

To prove this point, a 2005 survey published in one of the most prestigious scientific journals, *Nature*, exposed the inability of modern scientists to remain objective in the face of corporate pressures.[33] Questionable practices among researchers in the survey included the following:

• Falsifying or "cooking" research data
• Not properly disclosing conflicts of interest

- Failing to present contrary data

- Using inadequate or inappropriate research design

- Dropping observations or data points, and inadequate record keeping

The most alarming of the researchers' findings was that of the 3,247 scientists surveyed, *over 20 percent* admitted to changing the design, methodology, or results of a study in response to pressure from the funding source. The authors also noted that these numbers could be a gross underestimate of actual violations, since misbehaving scientists may have been less likely than others to respond to the survey for fear of discovery.

When science stands in the way of profits, corporations spare no expense at manipulating the facts. A classic example of this was the tobacco industry paying over $150,000 to a dozen scientists to "write" letters for publication in influential medical journals. The scientists did not actually write the letters themselves; they were written by lawyers for the tobacco industry. The doctors just signed them.[34]

After obtaining the letters published in reputable journals, the tobacco companies were then able to repeatedly cite the letters in defense of tobacco. Others assumed that the letters were written by independent scientists voicing their opinion. This is far from the only time that falsified independent third-party endorsements have been used as a public relations strategy.[35]

Third-Party Endorsements

Suppose I told you that I was selling a new vitamin that would make you feel fifteen years younger and could reverse almost any chronic disease. My product could make you stronger and improve your memory, intelligence, and looks. Would you believe me?

Even if you did, in a very short time the FDA would shut me down for making false claims; but even if it took them awhile to catch this, most people would view these claims with a healthy dose of skepticism. Educated consumers have learned that product manufacturers, regardless of the industry, will inflate the truth and manipulate information if it will help sell their products. Everyone has been exposed to advertising for products that will allow you to "shed pounds without exercise or diet" or "make you look and feel years younger."

Now imagine the same claims were made by important researchers who had no apparent financial connection to the vitamin. Doctors carrying impressive credentials announced that they had astounding results using this wonderful new formula. Additionally, a panel of certified government nutrition experts, such as the International Committee on Nutrition Excellence, had approved and endorsed the product.

You would likely be far more willing to accept these outlandish claims because an objective, independent, and respected third party endorses them.

Public-relations experts are well aware that third-party endorsements wield enormous influence. Business school students are routinely taught that third-party endorsements are so effective that, in many cases, they will actually increase sales figures more than advertisements. In the field of nutrition, third-party endorsements are commonplace. They often come from professional nutrition associations, or high-profile physicians or nutritionists.

Marketing experts have perfected the art of influencing (or in some case writing) statements that are used by "independent" experts. These statements are carefully worded and spoon-fed to the various media organizations to ensure that the intended corporate message is reaching the public. The media obligingly contributes to the corporate public deception by spreading word of the third-party endorsement, usually verbatim.

The artificial sweetener industry is no stranger to third-party endorsements. The media is loaded with seemingly important people such as Lyn Nabors, executive vice president of the Calorie Control Council, making statements such as, "Low-calorie sweeteners such as sucralose and the products that contain it offer people a way to manage calories without sacrificing taste. Using reduced calorie, sugar-free foods and beverages are directly in line with the recommendations of the 2005 Dietary Guidelines from the U.S. Department of Agriculture (USDA)."[36]

Most consumers do not realize that the Calorie Control Council is an association that represents the low-calorie, low-fat, and light food and beverage industry. The sole purpose of this organization is to represent over sixty manufacturers and suppliers that include McNeil Nutritionals, The NutraSweet Company, Proctor & Gamble (Olestra), Tate & Lyle, Sweet'N Low, Hershey's, The Coca-Cola Company, Abbot Laboratories (cyclamate), PepsiCo Inc., and more.

Endorsements from organizations such as the Calorie Control Council and others are delivered to the public as news. The media does not investigate possible conflicts of interest, nor does the public. These endorsements are taken at face value. There is rarely a balanced news article that equally portrays the opinion of those who are concerned about the safety record of artificial sweeteners along with the industry standpoint.

Can the Food Industry Buy Endorsements?

In an ideal perfect world, one could trust endorsements by nutritional organizations and societies. In addition to the Calorie Control Council, there are several highly visible nonprofit organizations including the American Council on Science and Health and the American Dietetics Association that promote themselves as independent voices of knowledge and reason in the nutrition field. Critics of these organizations are suspicious of their consistent and unwavering support of the food industry's agenda. You probably are not surprised to learn that these aforementioned organizations rely almost exclusively on food-industry financing to function.[37]

The American Council on Science and Health (ACSH) is promoted as a "consumer education organization concerned with issues related to food, nutrition, chemicals, pharmaceuticals, lifestyle, the environment, and health."[38] Its executive director regularly writes opinion editorials in highly visible media such as the *New York Times*, discussing the position the council takes on a variety of issues. The ACSH has enthusiastically defended virtually every chemical food additive backed by a major corporate interest. Not surprisingly, it has been reported that the ACSH receives over 75 percent of its funding from corporations and the rest from private foundations.[39]

The actions of the ACSH exemplify the abuse of third-party endorsements by the food industry. In an article published by former White House spokesman Betsy Hart titled "Irradiation Best Way to End E. Coli Threat," Elizabeth Whelan, the director of ACSH, says, "In fact, irradiation does wonderful things for a host of different foods . . . the unpopularity of irradiation to date in the United States is not based in science, but is due to anti-technology advocates who circulate unfounded claims that it poses a health hazard."[40]

The article makes no mention of opposing scientific viewpoints, of which there are many. In my opinion, this whole article is a gross example of an devious attempt to shape public opinion—a one-sided piece authored by a public-relations expert who uses the most controversial scientific opinions in the field to support her arguments. It is my guess that Hart did not write this article out of her personal and earnest concerns over E. coli in meat.

The ACSH's list of supporters consists of the usual suspects, including DuPont, Dow Chemicals, Frito-Lay, G. D. Searle, Hershey Foods Corp., Monsanto, Nestle, The NutraSweet Company, Coca-Cola, Johnson & Johnson, Kraft, Pepsi-Cola, Pfizer, and more.

Another suspiciously proindustry organization is the American Dietetic Association. The ADA blends mixed dietary advice with advertising, all the while, I would argue, providing diabetics with nutritional misinformation. For example, Dr. Richard Kahn, the ADA's chief scientific and medical officer, was quoted as saying, "There is not a shred of evidence that sugar has anything to do with getting diabetes."

He also said, "I don't think that there is any artificial sweetener on the market that has been shown to be unsafe."[41]

These astonishing statements are easily explained when you examine the corporate backing of the ADA. They certainly do not want to offend the people who are paying their salary and funding their organization.

The ADA is also responsible for the creation of nutritional facts sheets that are used as public education tools. The "fact sheets" are authored by the public-relations staff of various food manufacturers. It is disclosed on the fact sheets that they are "sponsored." But the true culprits are still cleverly disguised. The indicated sponsor on the aspartame fact sheet is not the NutraSweet Company, but the Calorie Control Council. The fact that the Calorie Control Council represents the interests of NutraSweet is conveniently omitted. Apparently, corporate headquarters at NutraSweet are interested in maintaining the valuable illusion of independent third-party endorsements.

The aspartame fact sheet in question contains one-sided statements such as, "Aspartame makes available a wide variety of food and beverage choices for the person interested in maintaining a healthy lifestyle," and "Is aspartame safe? Yes." There is no mention anywhere of the safety concerns associated with aspartame consumption.[42]

Federal Nutrition Policy: A By-Product of Corporate Desires

Most people consider nutrition a personal matter. What many do not realize is that the government has a comprehensive and detailed nutrition policy, and like it or not, it affects what you eat. Government laws and regulations control and regulate nearly every aspect of food production, preservation, and labeling. The government also plays a central role in nutrition education and dietary recommendations.

In an ideal world, the government's food recommendations and nutritional education would be based on sound research. The truth of the matter is that decisions surrounding mass food production and consumption are frequently economically motivated. Decision makers in Congress, the FDA, and the White House are strongly influenced by the many and varied special interest groups within the food industry.

The food companies influence the government's food policies through their aggressive lobbying techniques. Lobbyists are consultants paid to influence government policies and actions to favor their clients. In theory, lobbyists provide scientific advice that is pertinent to proposed regulations, industry-related legislation, and public education. In practice, lobbying usually includes arranging campaign contributions, drumming up favorable media, and exploiting social connections. Most lobbyists are ex-politicians who use their influence at social events, such as dinner parties, golf games, and cocktail hours to help advance their client's agenda.

Government agencies such as the FDA, USDA, and U.S. Agriculture Department are loaded with ex-lobbyists. The converse is true as well; many lobbyists are ex-government employees or politicians. You'll recall from previous chapters figures such as Donald Rumsfeld and Dr. Arthur Hayes Jr. alternating positions between government and industry, and providing privileged favors in each sector along the way. This merry-go-round of changing positions is common practice in the industry.

Attorney Michael Taylor began his law career as an FDA attorney, then transferred to a law firm representing food biotech giant Monsanto. Immediately following his career with Monsanto, Taylor returned to a government job as the deputy commissioner of policy at the FDA. Here, Taylor acted as part of a group that approved the use of Monsanto's genetically engineered growth hormone in cows. Taylor then moved on to the USDA as administrator for the food safety and inspection services. Finally, Taylor came full circle and returned to work for Monsanto as vice president for public policy. How can your health be protected when such conflicts of interest are pervasive in the government?

Those who support the current system feel that checks and balances are in place to prevent powerful industries from "buying" the support of government agencies. They also argue that it's all fair play, because lobbying is available to groups on both sides of any issue. But food and chemical industries have vastly superior funding and resources at their disposal.

Chemical manufacturers introduce thousands of new chemicals into our environment each year. And for each one, they need the government's approval to do so. From 1998 to 2005, drugmakers spent $758 million on lobbying politicians.[43] The goal of corporate lobbying is to influence what food and drug products can be marketed and how they are labeled. In the 2004 elections alone, nearly $17 million was contributed to political campaigns, including $1 million to President George W. Bush, and over $100,000 each to eighteen members of Congress. The drug industry employs 1,274 full-time lobbyists just for Washington, D.C., including forty former members of Congress.[44] These corporate lobbyists are extremely successful at what they do, which is putting the FDA at the mercy of the very same industries they aim to regulate.

Major international food corporations have frequently opposed policies that would promote sound nutrition advice. Marion Nestle, author of *Food Politics*, sheds some light on how food-industry influence on public policy is often counterproductive to improving nutrition. As the managing editor of the 1988 Surgeon General's Report on Nutrition and Health, Nestle experienced firsthand how food industry lobbyists will directly block potential advancements in public health if it could mean a loss in profits.

The 1988 Surgeon General's Report on Nutrition and Health was designed to be the first comprehensive review of research exploring the links between diet and chronic disease. Lobbyists from every food category visited Washington, D.C., before its publication, and all were very curious what the document would say. As the managing editor, Nestle was stunned when she was informed of one of the fundamental rules for writing the report: no matter what the research findings were, the report could not advise consumers to eat less beef, dairy, or any other category of food that was well represented by lobbyists. The reason for the rules was simple: if any information in the report adversely affected any of the major food industries, that industry would complain to Congress and the report would be lost in congressional debates—never to be seen again.[45]

The Surgeon General's Report could have been an objective, eye-opening research document that served as a dietary wake-up call for Americans. Instead, the final product was an industry-friendly report with watered-down dietary advice.

The United States Department of Agriculture's (USDA) Dietary Guidelines have been similarly influenced by corporate interests. Most nutritional experts disagreed with the *Eating Right Pyramid* the USDA released in 1991 because it was based on heavy pressure from food-industry lobbyists instead of proper nutrition. In fact, the publication of the *Eating Right Pyramid* was delayed for an entire year due to the protests of the National Cattlemen's Association, which felt that the *Pyramid* did not recommend enough beef. The advisory committee that revised the Dietary Guidelines in 2000 was riddled with rampant conflict of interest; of its eleven members, six had affiliations to the dairy, egg, and meat industries.[46]

Can the FDA Protect You from Corporate Greed?

What you've read so far should give you ample justification to question any manufacturer who has funded the frequently self-serving studies that verify the safety of the product they are selling—especially one that will ultimately wind up in your body.

But perhaps it's irrelevant that you simply can't trust the manufacturers of artificial sweeteners; after all, isn't there a federal regulatory and safety agency designed to protect you from their greed? The majority of people believe that artificial sweeteners are safe because the FDA has approved them. However, those who understand the function—and dysfunction—of the FDA know better than to blindly take their word on safety.

In the next chapter, I'll show you how the FDA has been completely subverted by the very industry they are intended to regulate—an industry that now calls the shots regarding what tests are appropriate to determine safety, and how safety is defined in the first place.

CHAPTER SIX:
SWEET DEALS

BIG BUSINESS AND THE FDA

The FDA is probably the most powerful federal regulatory agency, as it supervises over $1 trillion worth of products every year in the United States. To put this into perspective, the FDA has some form of influence on one quarter of every dollar you spend. The FDA's mandate is to certify that food, medicine, medical devices, cosmetics, and many other kinds of products are safe and effective. The FDA also regulates food and drug labeling and advertising.

The FDA's decisions have an enormous impact on the American economy, and anything that affects the American economy on such a large scale has the potential to become highly political. That's one of the primary reasons why the drug companies have the most powerful political lobby in Washington, with two lobbyists for every congressman.

The FDA and Artificial Sweeteners

The FDA has been given the responsibility to administer the certification of all sugar substitutes, including nonnutritive sweeteners, artificial sweeteners, and noncaloric sweeteners. As I mentioned earlier, the 1958 Food Additives Amendment to the Food, Drug, and Cosmetic Act governs the regulation of all sweeteners. According to the amendment, a sweetener can be considered safe in one of two ways:

1. It can be classified as Generally Recognized As Safe (GRAS). This GRAS list includes ingredients that were commonly used in foods before 1958, or ingredients that are judged by scientific evaluation to be safe to add directly or indirectly to food.

2. It can be approved through a food-additive petition, which requires comprehensive testing to establish the ingredient's safety and to establish an acceptable daily intake (ADI). The ADI is the amount of a food additive a person can safely consume on a daily basis over a lifetime.

Even insiders at the FDA recognize the approval process is far from perfect. As a consumer of American food and drugs, it has become vital to appreciate the deep impact of the manifold shortcomings of the FDA approval process. Manufacturers of artificial sweeteners hide behind FDA approval like it's a bulletproof vest. They treat FDA approval like an impenetrable shield that protects them from any potential safety concerns, both present and future, that were raised during the approval process. Whenever deleterious health associations or links to cancer are questioned, manufacturers consistently defend their product by arguing that the FDA has carefully examined these issues and determined there is no associated risk. The FDA typically backs up the manufacturer with reassuring statements, which is enough to bolster public confidence, pacify the media, and maintain or increase sales.

For example, the FDA has a 2004 review of the safety of artificial sweeteners on their Web site, FDA.gov, which stated, "There is no evidence that the regulated artificial sweeteners on the market in the United States are related to cancer risk in humans."[1]

Meanwhile, researchers at the University of Cologne in Germany published the following in the *Annals of Oncology*: "Case-control studies showed an elevated relative risk of 1.3 for heavy artificial sweetener use (no specific substances specified) of >1.7 g/day. For new generation sweeteners, it is too early to establish any epidemiological evidence about possible carcinogenic risks."[2]

It certainly sounds like the FDA has a distorted interpretation of available data. An agency whose founding mission was public safety might have a more cautionary tone to the public about artificial sweeteners. The FDA could tell the public that it's premature to say whether or not artificial sweeteners carry an increased risk of cancer. Instead, they're telling you that they are safe for everyone. While they do, studies continue to come out like those mentioned in chapter 3, linking aspartame to leukemia and lymphomas in animal studies. But the FDA continues to ignore such studies, cling to their earlier interpretations based on highly conflicted industry funded data, and issue misleading public reassurances.

Opinion polls show that people perceive the FDA as their trustworthy protector, performing an important regulatory function. But recalls and safety concerns over drugs like Vioxx, Crestor, Celebrex, Bextra, Meridia, Serevant, Mibefradil, Fen-Phen, Terfenadine, Bromfenac, Troglitazone, and others have opened a Pandora's box full of questions about serious conflicts of interest that virtually assure that the FDA will fail to fulfill its mandate.

How Did the FDA Acquire Its Vast Powers?

At the beginning of the twentieth century, food and medicine production were uncontrolled territories. Corruption, exploitation, and fraud were rampant. When Upton Sinclair documented the unsanitary conditions of the meatpacking industry in his 1906 book *The Jungle*, it shocked the world. This, combined with public disclosures about ineffective and dangerous medicines, led to the enactment of the Food and Drug Administration Act of 1906. This act prohibited the sale of misbranded and adulterated food, drinks, or drugs. It also signified the birth of the FDA, then called the Bureau of Chemistry.

However, this early form of the organization had very little power, so corruption and exploitation continued unchecked. But over the years, disasters and tragedies triggered structural changes that strengthened the FDA's regulatory powers.

In 1937, a well-intentioned chemist developed the "elixir sulfanilamide," a liquid form of sulfanilamide intended as a children's medication for sore throats. Diethylene glycol, also known as antifreeze, was used in the product.

The law at this time did not require that manufacturers prove their product was safe, and 240 gallons of the elixir were released into the marketplace.

This tragedy led to 107 accidental deaths. Congress, in response, enacted the Federal Food, Drug, and Cosmetic Act of 1938, which is considered the transition to the modern FDA. This act gave the FDA more power and control, and required the manufacturer (but not the FDA) to prove the safety of a product before it could be marketed.

The thalidomide catastrophe of the late 1950s triggered yet another amendment to the Federal Food, Drug, and Cosmetic Act. Thalidomide was heavily marketed in Europe as a sedative and sleeping pill. It also caused significant nerve damage and birth defects. The first of many "thalidomide babies" was born in Germany in 1958. These grossly deformed babies had no bones in their arms or legs. The hands and feet came directly from the trunk and were given the term *seal limbs*. In addition, the children often had no bowel opening, no ear openings, and a segmented colon.

Thalidomide manufacturers denied any problems with the drug. They said that the associations between the drug and birth defects were purely speculative, and they discredited physicians who sought to warn the public of the potential danger.

The FDA was in the process of evaluating thalidomide when its grave side effects first became evident. Over one thousand physicians in the United States were already prescribing thalidomide as part of the preapproval testing. The usual corruption and coercion by the manufacturer (in this case a subsidiary of Vick Chemical Company, known for Vick's VapoRub®) downplayed the dangers of thalidomide during the approval process.

The manufacturers of thalidomide continued to put pressure on the FDA for approval, threatening lawsuits, complaining to Congress, and harassing physicians who were reporting side effects. But the FDA prevailed and did not approve thalidomide. Instead it sent out FDA investigators to confiscate more than 2.5 million thalidomide tablets, unlabeled tablets, liquids, and powders that had been distributed in the United States.

When the truth about thalidomide became apparent to the general public, the FDA was hailed as saving America from the catastrophe that had hit Europe. The event stimulated the government to give the FDA even more regulatory power, such as a 1962 amendment that forced manufacturers to prove that not only was a drug safe, but it was also effective for the claims made on the label. Drug effectiveness had to be shown through sound scientific investigations led by qualified professionals.

The FDA was firmly established in the public eye as a trustworthy and necessary organization. And in fact, the early changes and amendments that molded the FDA all made very good sense. Laws and policies were geared toward creating a regulatory agency that could ensure public safety.

But change seems to be one of the virtual certainties of life, and the regulatory power of the FDA was no exception to this inevitability.

Big Pharma Uses HIV to Influence FDA Changes

Starting in 1987, controversial changes to FDA policies began to pave the way for greater influence by drug companies. The HIV crisis of the eighties put serious pressures on the FDA for faster approval of new drugs to combat this potential pandemic. Congress was convinced that the goal of protecting the public from unsafe and useless drugs conflicted with the goal of developing and introducing new drugs quickly. Public outcry grew over the lack of available drugs already on the market in other countries. There was a significant push from pharmaceutical companies for faster approval times.

Congress was pressured to accelerate the drug-approval process, but they knew the FDA did not have the budget or staff to move any faster. Congress concluded that the best solution was to create a partnership. They advised the FDA to work closely with the drug companies to decrease the time it took to approve drugs. President Clinton encouraged FDA department chiefs to view the drugmakers as "partners" instead of "adversaries."

But this new position failed to factor in the extensive history of massive corruption and conflict of interest that was pervasive in the industry and its potential to pervert the FDA regulatory process. Congressional supporters of this new legislation created the image that drug companies were research institutions well-intentioned for the public good and benefactors of the human race. It was if the dark side of the pharmaceutical industry had somehow never existed and somehow magically disappeared.

Supporters of new legislation to speed up drug approval, such as Robert Goldberg of the Manhattan Institute, felt that getting valuable technology to the public required a more rapid turnaround. Goldberg stated that the FDA is a cumbersome bureaucratic agency that "protects the people from drugs that can save their lives."[3] Goldberg suggested that the FDA's role should be shifted to get drugs into the marketplace as quickly as possible, and monitor their impact after marketing rather than wait for needless clinical trials.

But the motivation for speedy approval for new pharmaceuticals is rarely to provide lifesaving drugs to the public. The conventional medical system is largely based on the drug-for-profit model. Now I don't think it is immoral for a drug company to make a profit. However, I am strongly opposed to a system where people's lives are ruined as a result of this reckless pursuit for maximum profits. As you will see very shortly, this appears to be the case for a large number of drugs that the FDA initially approved but were eventually removed from the market.

Additionally, very few drugs are researched and developed to treat diseases like malaria, which kills millions of people worldwide—but mostly poor people. Those types of medicines, when they are financed at all, are subsidized by governments or wealthy philanthropists like Bill Gates, rather than private industries. Drug companies are constantly searching for blockbuster drugs like Viagra, Lipitor, and Prozac that can be mass-marketed at a high price and used for long periods of time, leading to windfall profits. When examined more carefully, it becomes obvious that the real goal of the accelerated approval process is to maximize the usable life span of a patent for a maximum return on investment for Big Pharma.

You may not realize that patents for new drugs are issued well before a drug reaches the market. The time period between a patented drug's approval and patent expiration is considered the company's profit window. The life of a patent is twenty to twenty-five years, and a long approval process can leave only five to ten years of exclusive marketing rights. The sooner a drug is brought to market, the longer the company has to bring in profit before less expensive generic brands erase their profit margins.

Over time, the drug lobbyists prevailed, and new regulations were developed to expedite drug approval, which lowered the standards and allowed drugs to be approved without a comprehensive investigation. But rather than providing you with better and more innovative lifesaving drugs, the major change appears to have been an enormous improvement in the drug companies' bottom lines; a 2002 study estimated that of all the drugs approved for the prior decade, only 15 percent were made of new ingredients that provided significant clinical benefit over drugs already on the market.[4]

Dr. David Graham, who is the associate director for Science and Medicine in the Office of Drug Safety with the FDA, has estimated that about two-thirds to three-quarters of the drugs that the FDA reviews are already on the market and are being reviewed for another indication.

Fast Times at the FDA

The approval time for new drugs was eventually shortened by approximately two years. Now the average time for a new drug to complete the process is only twelve months, and a mere six months for drugs considered to be a high priority. Every day a drug is held up from being marketed represents a loss of one million to two million dollars of profit. It wasn't long before manufacturers took full advantage of this new treasure chest of opportunity. The number of applications for new approvals grew faster than the staff or budget of the FDA could possibly handle. This led to the most controversial policy change in the history of the FDA, the Prescription Drug User Fee Act of 1992.

The Prescription Drug User Fee Act allows the FDA to collect "user fees" from drug companies. The user fees are used to help fund the FDA by increasing their resources for approval process. These fees now account for half of the FDA's budget for drug evaluation, and 12 percent of the agency's overall $1.3 billion budget. The problem is that now that the FDA is dependent on the food and drug companies for their funding, many people at the FDA are reluctant to bite the hand that feeds them.

In a recent interview, Dr. David Graham shared his views on how this legislation has affected the FDA:

> As currently configured, the FDA is not able to adequately protect the American public. It's more interested in protecting the interests of industry. It views industry as its client, and the client is someone whose interest you represent. Unfortunately, that is the way the FDA is currently structured. Within the Center for Drug Evaluation and Research, about 80 percent of the resources are geared towards the approval of

new drugs and 20 percent is for everything else. Drug safety is about 5 percent.[5]

The Fox Is Guarding the Henhouse

The User Fee Act forged a deadly partnership between the FDA and the pharmaceutical industry. The FDA now receives corporate sponsorship from the very industry it was created to regulate. The FDA has gone from watchdog of the pharmaceutical industry to its lapdog. A myriad of FDA activities in the past few years reveal the FDA's willingness to serve the agenda of the multibillion-dollar pharmaceutical giants.

Prior to the act, only 4 percent of new drugs were submitted to the FDA for approval before any other world agency. But in 1998, they were first to approve 66 percent of new drugs. And prior to the 1992 legislation, the FDA only approved 60 percent of the drugs presented to the agency. By the end of the nineties, though, 80 percent of applications were approved. Congress and the drug companies are very pleased with the new system, but this satisfaction comes at the expense of public safety.

The User Fee Act has jeopardized public confidence in the FDA's ability to maintain objectivity. Busy physicians who rely on the FDA to monitor new drugs for safety now find themselves wondering how careful an evaluation has actually been performed and what has been conveniently swept under the rug.

Just when it seemed things couldn't get worse, in 1997 the Food and Drug Modernization Act was enacted. This legislation extended User Fees and further lowered the already-weakened standard approval process for drugs. Some drugs can now be approved after only one clinical trial. It also expanded the use of accelerated approvals. And the Modernization Act lifted the ban on allowing the marketing of drugs for non-FDA approved uses. Off-label use marketing has opened a whole new flow of income for drug companies.

> Did you know that the research shows the modern health-care system is the leading cause of death? Dr. Gary Null and others conducted a $50,000 study that definitively analyzed peer-reviewed journals and government health statistics and reached this startling conclusion. I have a summary of his groundbreaking work complete with tables and statistics on my Web site.[6]

Deadly FDA Approved Drugs

The following is a sampling of drugs approved by the FDA that have caused severe injury or death:

Baycol, manufactured by Bayer, is a cholesterol-lowering statin drug taken by 700,000 Americans—and was pulled off the market in 2001. It had been linked to thirty-one U.S. deaths from a severe muscle disorder called rhabdomyolysis (a large number of skeletal muscle cells die). At least nine more fatalities abroad are known.

Bextra, manufactured by Pfizer, is a specific kind of nonsteroidal anti-inflammatory drug known as a Cox-2 inhibitor used for pain conditions such as arthritis. It was withdrawn in 2005 for doubling the risk of heart attacks and strokes.

Cylert, manufactured by Abbott, is a central nervous system stimulant for the treatment of Attention Deficit Hyperactivity Disorder (ADHD). To date, the FDA has received thirteen reports of Cylert-associated liver failure leading to liver transplantation or death. Although the manufacturer, Abbott, has ceased the sales and marketing of Cylert, it remains on the market with a warning label.

Duract, manufactured by Wyeth-Ayerst, is a painkiller, approved despite FDA medical investigators' warnings of severe liver toxicity. Duract is suspected in sixty-eight deaths due to liver failure. It was on the market for less than a year and recalled in 1998.

Hismanal-D, manufactured by Janssen LP (owned by Johnson & Johnson), is an antihistamine taken for allergies. Approved in 1988 and soon known to cause cardiac arrhythmias, the drug was finally taken off the market in 1999.

Lotronex, manufactured by GlaxoSmithKline (GSK), is a drug for treating irritable bowel syndrome in women, approved by the FDA administrators despite warnings from investigating FDA medical officers and preapproval evidence of severe side effects. The drug is reported to cause life-threatening intestinal inflammation called ischemic colitis, constipation so severe that some patients require removal of parts of their intestines, severely obstructed or ruptured bowels (complications of severe constipation), and death (five deaths so far). GSK voluntarily withdrew the drug from the market in 2001 but then put it back on the market after creating a "risk management program" that includes a black box warning and a patient consent form.

Palladone, manufactured by Purdue Pharma LP is a narcotic for pain. It was approved in 2004, but the FDA asked Purdue to withdraw it in 2005 due to possible fatal side effects when taken with alcohol.

Pondimin, manufactured by Wyeth-Ayerst, is an appetite suppressant and a component of Fen-Phen, the diet fad drug. Approved in 1973, Pondimin's link to heart valve damage and a lethal pulmonary disorder wasn't recognized until shortly before its withdrawal in 1997.

Posicor, manufactured by Roche, a blood pressure medication, was approved by the FDA in 1997 despite preapproval evidence that it can fatally disrupt heart-beat rhythm. It was also shown to have potentially fatal interactions with over twenty-five other commonly prescribed medications. Posicor showed no special benefit when compared to previously available blood pressure medications. Posicor is suspected in over a hundred deaths. Roche recalled the drug in 1998.

Propulsid, manufactured by Janssen Pharmaceuticals, is medication for severe nighttime heartburn, approved in 1993 despite evidence that it can cause heart rhythm irregularities, heart attacks, and sudden death. At least 341 reports of heart-rhythm abnormalities, including 80 reports of deaths, have been associated with Propulsid. The drug was allowed to remain on the market for an additional six months after initial withdrawal. The FDA claimed it was to give patients time to switch to alternative therapies. This decision conveniently coincided with Johnson & Johnson's new heartburn drug, Aciphex, becoming available. Janssen pulled it off the market in 2000.

Raxar, manufactured by GSK, is an antibiotic and was approved in 1997 despite heart-rhythm disturbances and deaths in preapproval clinical trials. The FDA did not require any warnings on the product insert for the problems found in the clinical trials. Two years and eighteen deaths later, GSK voluntarily recalled Raxar from the market.

Redux, manufactured by Wyeth-Ayerst, is an appetite suppressant and a component of Fen-Phen, the diet fad drug. It was approved despite the FDA advisory board voting against the drug. The FDA analyzed heart tests on 291 dieters and found almost a third—92 people—had damaged heart valves, even though they had no symptoms. Redux is suspected in 123 deaths. The FDA asked Wyeth to withdraw the drug in 1997.

Rezulin, manufactured by Warner-Lambert, a diabetes drug, approved in 1997 despite a FDA medical officer (Dr. David Graham) presenting strong and unambiguous evidence of liver toxicity in preapproval trials. Rezulin is suspected in 391 deaths. The drug wasn't taken off the market until 2000.

Seldane, manufactured by Hoechst Marion Roussel, and approved in 1985, was world's top-selling allergy medication for a decade despite the side effects that included cardiac arrhythmias, blackouts, hospitalizations, and deaths. Only after the FDA approved their new allergy drug, Allegra-D, did Hoechst agree to remove Seldane from the market in 1997.

Tysabri, manufactured by Biogen Idec Inc. and Elan Corp., was expected to become the world's leading treatment for MS when it was approved in 2004. However, after three patients developed PML (progressive multifocal leukoencephalopathy), of which two died, the drug was withdrawn. PML is a rare but serious viral infection of the brain. In June 2006, the FDA reapproved the drug.

Vioxx, manufactured by Merck, is a specific kind of nonsteroidal anti-inflammatory drug known as a Cox-2 inhibitor used for pain conditions such as arthritis. Preapproval data showed a sevenfold increase risk for heart attacks with low-dose Vioxx, but the FDA approved it anyway. Vioxx is suspected in 160,000 cases of heart attacks and strokes in the United States alone. On September 2004, Merck voluntarily recalled Vioxx after a study was released that showed increased heart-attack risk. In Feburary 2005, the FDA voted 17–15 to return Vioxx to the market, but Merck has not done so as it is occupied with all of its lawsuits.

FUN FACT:

Nearly twenty million patients (almost 10 percent of the U.S. population) were exposed to five drugs that were recalled in 1997 and 1998 alone.

The most troubling aspect of these drug approvals is that these drugs were not lifesaving wonder drugs. They were for treating conditions such as weight loss, high blood pressure, diabetes, and pain. Many of these drugs were "me too" drugs, minimally modified biochemical clones of ones already on the market, but sold by a different manufacturer. They did not represent any note-worthy advances in therapy. In all cases there were other, safer drugs to treat these conditions already available. There was absolutely no reason, other than increased drug company profits, not to conduct thorough evaluations of these drugs before making them available.

Record Number of Drugs Required Removal from the Market

Never before has the FDA withdrawn so many drugs in such a short period of time.[7] With each new drug withdrawal, it becomes more and more evident that the drug approval process is indeed a prescription for disaster. FDA officials have been so desperate to deflect the responsibility that they resorted to publishing an analysis of their own work. In 1999, the *Journal of the American Medical Association* published an FDA assessment that reached the bizarre conclusion that accelerated drug approval is totally unrelated to the increase in dangerous drugs being withdrawn. Their conclusion was that there are more drugs, more applications for approval, and the population is on more medication than ever before; therefore, the increase in recalls is a natural consequence.

Would you possibly expect any other conclusion when the fox is guarding the henhouse?

FDA—Foisting Drugs on America

An internal FDA report in 2002 found that one-third of FDA employees were not comfortable challenging data supplied by drug companies.[8] When a reviewer raises concern about a drug's safety, his or her actions are stigmatized. FDA scientists are shown that they must play the game or step to the sidelines. The FDA has shifted to making its decisions based on corporate mandates rather than objective impartial science. The FDA has changed from asking *if they should* approve drugs to *how they will* approve them.[9]

As an example of the indefensible position the FDA has shifted to, consider Dr. Michael Elashoff, PhD. Elashoff was an FDA advisor assigned to approve a new flu drug, Relenza. Elashoff, a well-trained biostatistician from Harvard, concluded there was no proof Relenza worked. His presentation to the advisory panel stated that patients would be exposed to risk without deriving any benefit. An agency advisory committee denied approval of Relenza by a vote of thirteen to four. This was not what senior officials wanted to hear. Elashoff was quickly removed from the advisory panel of a second flu drug and told he would no longer make presentations to the advisory committee. Meanwhile, Relenza was approved as a safe and effective flu drug.

This is typical of many cases when medical advisors determine that a drug is unsafe or ineffective and dismissed because their findings conflict with the drug companies' data. Reviewers can be demoted for merely seeking to abide by the Hippocratic Oath: "First do no harm." FDA senior officials put pressure on reviewers to approve new drugs, and put obstacles and hurdles in the way of disapproving a drug. Investigators who choose to diligently perform their job even when it conflicts with the drug company agenda may face serious consequences. The FDA has morphed into an agency of highly educated and well-intentioned physicians and scientists who are practically handcuffed from effectively doing their jobs.

FDA officials are pressured by the drug companies and Congress. The FDA has become dependent on the pharmaceutical industry for most of its funding, and the drug companies complain to Congress if their drugs are not rapidly and consistently approved. The $100 billion pharmaceutical industry, which has contributed hundreds of millions of dollars to politicians in the past few years alone, has no problem getting the government's undivided attention. FDA leaders are concerned that lengthy approval times or higher drug denial rates will upset Congress. Congress could in turn lash back and withdraw user fees, which would devastate the FDA's operating budget and cost thousands of jobs.

Corporate Sponsorship of the FDA—
Just the Tip of the Iceberg

The Prescription Drug Users Act and the Modernization Act has led to a new policy at the FDA: don't bite the hand that feeds you. Pressure for fast-paced approval, in an environment that discourages raising concerns about the investigational drugs, creates a sweatshop environment for many FDA employees. Reviewers are often presented with truckloads of data, given a completely unreasonable time to evaluate all of it, and then discouraged from reaching their own conclusions.

FDA reviewers are highly trained and educated researchers, but they are still human. The current climate at the FDA is causing an unacceptable amount of employee burnout. In 2002, the *Wall Street Journal* reported that 15 percent of FDA medical officer jobs were vacant. FDA employee turnover is significantly higher than at other government agencies such as the NIH and the CDC.[10] A recent survey mailed to nearly six thousand FDA scientists found that nearly 40 percent of them believe the agency is not acting effectively to protect the public health.[11]

Top scientists who have committed their lives to public safety are in a system that has evolved into handicapping them from properly performing their assignments, and this conflict is creating enormous stress and tension. Honest scientists reluctantly contribute to approval of dubious drugs, or, in some cases, drugs are approved against the investigators' recommendations. Then their hands are tied as they watch these same drugs harm thousands of people.[12]

Massive Conflict of Interest on Advisory Panels

The responsibility of FDA officers is to report their interpretations of thousands of pages of drug company data to one of the agency's eighteen advisory panels. FDA advisory panels are designed to consist of experts from the appropriate medical community. They are chartered to use their expertise to advise the government on the safety and effectiveness of medicine. Federal law prevents the FDA from hiring experts with any potential conflicts of interest. However, between 1998 and 2000, the FDA waived this restriction more than eight hundred times.[13] It has been estimated that over half of all advisory panels have financial ties to the pharmaceutical companies that stand to gain or lose from their decision.

The FDA's deadly partnership with the pharmaceutical industry has permeated all levels of drug approval. After safety questions were raised about the controversial COX-2 painkillers (Vioxx, Celebrex, and Bextra), an FDA advisory panel met in 2005 and agreed to allow COX-2 drugs to remain on the market. The Center for Science in the Public Interest hired the *New*

York Times to investigate any possible conflict of interest, and they found that one-third of the panel had ties to the very drug company they were seeking to regulate. If the votes of these individuals were removed, then the COX-2 inhibitors would not have been allowed to return to the market.[14] Despite the *New York Times'* exposé, the FDA has yet to overturn their decision, but fortunately for the public, as of the writing of this book Vioxx has not been reintroduced to the market.

FDA senior associate commissioner Linda Suydam, who is responsible for waiving conflict of interest restrictions, states that often the best experts to hire are the same experts who consult the industry.[15] Unfortunately this does not explain how "consumer representatives" on advisory panels often also have financial ties to the industry.

Who Provides the FDA with Safety Data?

The FDA drug approval process requires the manufacturer to provide animal studies that screen for pharmacological activity and toxicity potential. If the drug passes this stage, they are given approval to run their own clinical studies on humans. The problem with this system is that the FDA relies on the research done by the manufacturers that can be seriously biased. There is no requirement for research conducted by an unbiased independent party in this process.[16] This is fundamentally wrong and fatally flawed; it's yet another setup for massive conflict of interest and a prescription for disaster.

These sophisticated companies can easily manipulate their data, especially when they are seeking to conceal links to chronic diseases, such as cancer, heart disease, or diabetes. Researchers consistently skew, hide, or deny knowledge of such potential dangers to human health.

Currently, the FDA merely requires a summary of the manufacturer's research findings. All too often, these summaries gloss over indications of potential health hazards by stating the results were "inconclusive" or that they "were not able to establish a direct causative link."

What does this mean in plain language? Typically, it means that even though a significant number of animals or people in a study got sick or died, the manufacturers can misrepresent the facts and numbers so it cannot be "scientifically and statistically" proven that their product is responsible for the observed effect.

What do you expect? Corporations are mandated by law to put their stockholders interest first, so they will do what it takes to increase their profits. They are paying for the study and clearly want to present the best possible picture to the FDA so their significant investment will be approved and the money will start rolling in.

Vioxx, Merck, and the FDA

That brings us back to Merck's blockbuster drug, Vioxx. The recent controversies surrounding this drug have eliminated any remaining doubt about who the FDA is really trying to protect.

Vioxx is a nonsteroidal, anti-inflammatory drug (NSAID) known as a selective COX-2 inhibitor. NSAIDs as a group are the most common cause of adverse drug reactions. Gastrointestinal bleeding, ulcers, and perforation caused by NSAIDs and aspirin are the main causes of hospital admissions resulting from legal drug use. In 1991, two COX-enzymes were discovered and designated COX-1 and COX-2. It was determined that COX-2 is largely responsible for blocking inflammation and COX-1 causes the harmful gastrointestinal symptoms associated with NSAID drugs. This started a race for drug companies to develop potential blockbuster NSAIDs with the benefits of COX-2 but none of the drawbacks of COX-1.

In 1999, Celebrex and Vioxx were the first two COX-2 inhibitors to hit the American market. As expected, these drugs were an instant success. But concerns over the safety of these drugs were immediate—NSAIDs in general are also known to have injurious effects on the cardiovascular system.

Prior to approval of Vioxx, Merck conducted a study named "090" that showed a sevenfold increase in heart-attack risk at low doses. The FDA approved Vioxx in May 1999. The labeling at approval said nothing about heart-attack risks.[17]

In November 2000, another Merck clinical trial named "VIGOR" found a fivefold increase in heart-attack risk at high doses. In spite of these alarming statistics, Merck insisted Vioxx was safe because the results were related to the heart-attack prevention effects of the control group taking naproxen rather than the cardiotoxic effects of Vioxx.[18] A serious challenge to this argument, though, was that naproxen had not been shown to have any previous heart-attack prevention effects. Merck results about three heart attacks among study participants before submitting the study to the *New England Journal of Medicine*. The editors of the *Journal* discovered the missing data in 2001 but did not suspect it was an intentional omission until 2005 when the lawsuits began.[19]

More and more Vioxx trials were published reporting an increased heart-attack risk with Vioxx use. In addition, it is estimated that since its approval, Vioxx has caused over 160,000 heart attacks and strokes.[20] As negative publicity grew from these reports, Merck was forced into damage-control mode, and on September 30, 2004, they removed Vioxx from the market. But by doing so, Merck also dodged recommendations from FDA safety officers to look into the potential cardiovascular risks. Instead, Merck was busy pumping its resources into research that would allow them to market Vioxx for other medical conditions.[21] Preliminary data from a study using Vioxx to prevent colon polyps revealed unambiguous evidence of increased risk of heart attack and stroke from the drug. Merck was initially praised for acting promptly to "new" evidence about the safety of Vioxx.

Merck was doing everything in its power to come out of this scandal looking good. But the magnitude of their greed did not make this possible. In 2004, investigations by the *Wall Street Journal* provided evidence that Merck was fully aware of Vioxx's risk as early as 2000. Internal documents revealed Merck had every intention of concealing Vioxx's risks from doctors and the public. The literature Merck used to train its sales representatives on how to respond to questions was titled *Dodge Ball Vioxx*. The authors of the *Wall Street Journal* article concluded that the drug should have been withdrawn from the market several years earlier. When Merck finally pulled the plug on Vioxx, their stock prices collapsed, and they lost about $30 billion in market value.[22, 23]

Something few expected to emerge from the Vioxx scandal was the full disclosure of the kind of corruption that brought Vioxx to the marketplace. But Dr. David Graham, associate director of the FDA's office of drug safety, did just that in his testimony before Congress. Dr. Graham is a twenty-year veteran of the FDA and a true scholar, educated at some of the leading medical schools in the world, including Johns Hopkins University School of Medicine and Yale University. Throughout Dr. Graham's career, he has been a steadfast advocate of drug safety at the FDA.

When Dr. Graham stood before the Senate committee, he took the opportunity to expose the current FDA structure as critically flawed. He told Congress that Vioxx was likely responsible for killing at least sixty thousand people from heart attacks and strokes. Instead of sweeping Vioxx under the rug as an isolated drug catastrophe, Graham also warned Congress of the FDA's systemic failure to properly weigh the risks and benefits of drugs. He divulged past FDA controversial oversights and exposed other unsafe drugs currently being consumed by Americans.[24] Dr. Graham, a man who knows what the FDA does and does not do, concluded that *the FDA's current structure is incapable of protecting Americans.* When it comes to drug and food safety, Americans are left to fend for themselves.

Four million Americans were taking Vioxx at the time of its withdrawal. As with many other dangerous drugs that make it to market, there were much safer, older drugs in the same category already available. Dangerous and overpriced drugs are filling pharmacy shelves, and we, the American health-care consumers, are paying the price.

CHANGES TO THE FDA TO INCREASE PUBLIC SAFETY ACCORDING TO DR. GRAHAM:

1. The FDA must be truly independent and transparent. The pharmaceutical industry cannot be a direct source of funding for the agency.

2. FDA advisory panels must be cleaned up. Financial conflicts of interest should never be allowed. All advisory panel members' financial affiliations should be public information.

3. New drugs and food additives should be introduced to the public with precautionary warnings. Minimal safety data does not equate to marketing that implies absolute safety. Aggressive marketing of new chemical compounds and encouraging widespread use in populations for which it is not tested is a dangerous exercise.

4. The FDA should be required to run a public awareness campaign that

---

> explains how most side effects of new chemical compounds remain undiscovered until after being consumed by the public for years.
>
> 5. The FDA must balance resources between review and approval of new drugs and food additives and obtaining postmarketing safety surveillance. The current structure is geared toward the approval process and "user's fees" are entirely dedicated to this process.
>
> 6. When safety concerns over a drug or food additive arise, an independent regulatory agency should investigate and take action. Once approval has been made, it is naturally in the approving agency's best interest to stand by its original decision.
>
> 7. Direct-to-consumer advertising for prescription drugs must end.[25]

In the wake of the Vioxx scandal, however, a glimpse of hope has emerged from within the greed and corruption that shapes the FDA. Dr. Graham has shown us that there are a few remaining FDA scientists whose moral character has survived the challenging environment of modern politics. You'll learn more about Dr. Graham's courageous testimony and sound advice for reforming the FDA in the next chapter. Scientists such as Dr. Graham remain committed to the goal of protecting Americans from useless and dangerous drugs and food products. These few remaining honest and dedicated scientists are the FDA's last chance to avoid completely becoming nothing more than a pawn of big business.

"Misinterpretation of the Data"

In June of 2006, the *New England Journal of Medicine* published another correction to this study that even further damaged Merck's position, "to make it completely clear" to their readers that eighteen months of Vioxx use is not necessary to increase heart risks. Heart risks from the painkiller, which was withdrawn from the market because of these concerns, can occur with just three months of use.

The *Wall Street Journal* believes that the correction could be a boon for those who have sued Merck, as this point was a cornerstone in Merck's defense. They persisted in stating that the drug could not damage anyone that had been on it for less than eighteen months. The correction could have major implications for the thirteen thousand lawsuits that allege Vioxx caused heart damage. At the correction date Merck has lost three cases and won three cases. In two of the cases that Merck won, the individuals had taken the drug less than eighteen months.[26]

Pharmaceutical Drugs Are One of the Leading Killers in the United States

FDA-approved drugs are killing record numbers of Americans, and the pattern appears to be getting worse instead of better. You probably aren't aware of this, as the Centers for Disease Control has conveniently determined that it will classify deaths on a pathological basis rather than a causal one. All sixty-thousand of the Vioxx related deaths are therefore classified as heart attacks, instead of classified as drug-induced death, concealing the truth.

Similarly, there are estimated to be over one hundred thousand non-error-related deaths due to pharmaceutical drugs every year in the United States. You can increase this by another third when you factor in accidental error-related deaths, such as when the physician prescribed the wrong drug or dose or the patient made an error. I believe these deaths are hidden and disguised in the current statistics to keep you in the dark as to just how dangerous the drug-based model truly is.

If you want to learn more about the life-threatening behavior of the pharmaceutical industry, you might want to take a look at *The Truth About the Drug Companies: How They Deceive Us and What to Do About It* by Marcia Angell, MD. As the executive editor of the *New England Journal of Medicine* for many years, Dr. Angell had a front-row seat for the appalling practices of the drug industry.

Competition Against Industry Interests, Like Stevia, Is Quickly Bashed by the FDA

An interesting contrast to the FDA's pattern of rapid approval and ignored health concerns that we have seen throughout this book is their treatment of the herb stevia. Stevia is the only natural sugar alternative that could compete with its synthetic counterparts. Because it's natural, it cannot be patented, and so has no chemical corporate interests to generate propaganda in favor of it. And it's also in the best interest of its competitors that it not be approved as a sweetening agent. The FDA's attitude toward it has differed accordingly.

Let's quickly review the potential dangers of artificial sweeteners, and the FDA response, which we have learned about in previous chapters:

Saccharin: Animal studies show it can cause cancer of the bladder. Saccharin has also caused cancer of the uterus, ovaries, skin, blood vessels, and other organs. It has been shown to increase the potency of other cancer-causing chemicals. Created early enough to be considered GRAS at first, it was not examined until independent non-FDA investigations brought the potential dangers to light. The FDA required a warning label on it for a while, but no longer does.

Cyclamate: Animal studies indicate it causes cancer and may increase the potency of other cancer-causing chemicals. A National Cancer Institute study found that heavy use of blended cyclamate and saccharin was associated with a higher incidence of bladder cancer. Like saccharin, it was created early enough to be considered GRAS at first, so it was likewise not examined until independent non-FDA investigations exposed the possible dangers. It has been banned by the FDA, but may be considered for reapproval.

Aspartame: Animal studies suggest aspartame is toxic to the nervous system. It was shown to cause damage to the brains of infant mice. Approved by the FDA, with a warning label required for those with PKU.

Sucralose: Preapproval data showed evidence for antifertility effects, immune system toxicity, potential mutagenic activity, and fetal edema in offspring. Approved by the FDA.

Acesulfame-K: Animal studies suggest it may cause cancer and breakdown products shown to be toxic to the thyroid gland. Approved by the FDA.

Neotame: Aspartame plus 3-di-methylbutyl, which can be found on the EPA's list of most hazardous chemicals. Approved by the FDA.

It's interesting to note how the more recent sweeteners, approved after the User Fee Act and the Food and Drug Modernization Act, sailed easily through the process even compared to the FDA's relatively friendly treatment of the earlier artificial sweeteners.

Now let's look at stevia. Stevia is a noncaloric herb, native to Paraguay, that has been used as a sweetener for centuries. While Japanese manufacturers have used stevia since the early 1970s to sweeten pickles and other foods, the FDA has turned down three industry requests to use stevia in foods in the United States. Stevia has been the subject of searches and seizures, trade complaints, and embargoes on importation. Supporters of stevia assert that FDA actions regarding stevia amount to a restraint to trade designed to benefit the artificial sweetener industry.

The FDA's treatment of petitions to approve stevia is quite interesting in light of their historically generous attitude toward synthetic chemical sweeteners. The general tone of the FDA is that stevia is an unsafe substance no matter how much evidence is provided to the contrary. Artificial sweeteners, as you have seen, are in contrast generally viewed as benign chemical compounds that are considered safe until there is a preponderance of research data to the contrary—and even then they may still be considered safe. Stevia is guilty until proven innocent; artificial sweeteners are innocent until proven guilty.

The Elimination of Stevia as a Sweetener: A Puzzling Paradox Explained by Politics

The issues surrounding stevia as a sweetener are undeniably political. Unfortunately for stevia, current politics are against it, and the FDA's actions appear to protect the health of big business rather than the health of the public. Backing artificial sweeteners are the global chemical giants Pfizer, Monsanto, Johnson & Johnson, Abbot Laboratories, and Hoechst. Petitioners for stevia include the American Herbal Products Association (AHPA) and the Lipton Tea Company. This is clearly an unbalanced battle.

A 1991 petition generated by the AHPA provided compelling evidence for stevia to receive GRAS status, which makes it exempt from the 1958 food additive provisions. We'll examine stevia's safety in greater detail in chapter 8, but for now it's enough to know that unequivocal evidence of widespread safe use by humans throughout history filled the pages of the AHPA petition. The FDA chose to ignore the unequivocal evidence; stevia was instead evaluated as a new food additive.

The petition voluntarily supplied scientific data, which is not even required because of stevia's common and widespread use pre-1958. The voluntary data included acute, subacute, carcinogenicity, and mutagenicity studies and evaluations. The cumulative data provided objective data that there are no safety problems associated with the use of stevia.

The FDA felt that the scientific data voluntarily submitted in the petitions was not enough. In 1994, the agency stated they did not have enough data to conclude that the use of stevia as a food additive would be safe. The FDA provided no explanation of why stevia would not be considered for GRAS status. Meanwhile, stevia makes up 40 percent of the Japanese sweetener market, and no reports of any adverse reactions have surfaced from thirty years of use in Japan.[27] (Contrast this with the fact that 80 percent of food-additive-related complaints in the United States are about aspartame, which the FDA has determined is safe.)

Since the passage of the Dietary Supplement Health and Education Act (DSHEA), stevia can be sold legally in the United States as a dietary supplement. It can be found in many forms. But it must be sold by itself, not incorporated into any product, and it must be labeled as a dietary supplement. Stevia cannot be called a sweetener or even referred to as sweet. To do so would violate FDA regulations and the product could be subject to seizure.

In the 1980s, an anonymous firm filed a trade complaint with the FDA about stevia. Celestial Seasonings, the herbal tea company, was using stevia at the time. They were ordered by the FDA to stop producing tea containing stevia. Traditional Medicinals, another tea company, had their inventory of stevia teas confiscated during an unexpected FDA raid. They were told that the tea would be destroyed. In another draconian action, the FDA ordered a Texas-based distributor of stevia supplements to destroy three books on the subject. In that case, the FDA's attempt at violating the First Amendment spurred public outrage, and the FDA decided not to follow through with the book burning.

Despite the Freedom of Information Act, the FDA will not reveal who made the trade complaint. Many are suspicious the complaint was filed by manufacturers of artificial sweeteners trying to fend off competition.

Throughout this book there are countless examples of preapproval data that suggested that artificial sweeteners carry a variety of risks. For each sweetener, the approval process included negotiations between the FDA and manufacturers. Studies that indicated health risks were redesigned and repeated to achieve the intended results. Other uncomplimentary data was deemed insignificant or inconclusive. Various committees went back and forth until the information could be sculpted into a clean bill of health.

The financial cost of the research necessary to look deeper into the studies for stevia is beyond the scope of an organization such as the American Herbal Products Association (AHPA). They don't have a relationship with the FDA like the multinational drug companies that help fund it, and which have worked closely with the FDA on thousands of approvals. Overall, the chances of stevia ever winning approval with the FDA as a sweetener are slim to none.

Stevia is a natural product, and there are no patent protections that allow exclusive rights to selling it. For these reasons, there are no corporations willing to make a financial investment into establishing the safety of stevia with the FDA (even though there are plenty of studies that already prove its safety). And now that stevia has been designated as unsafe, its designation is likely to remain unchanged. Experience shows that once the FDA has made a decision, it's highly unusual for them to reverse it, especially without pressure from big business. This is evident from the FDA's lack of response when it is time to remove dangerous drugs from the market, or withdraw hazardous food additives such as aspartame and Olestra.

Stevia has been consumed safely for over 1,500 years, and is processed from a plant that, coming from a natural source, makes it compatible with the human digestive system. Artificial sweeteners are new to the food supply, and are produced by large chemical companies who focus on inventing new compounds and selling them as food and drugs for a significant profit, with little attention to the long-term consequences to your health.

When it comes down to a choice between trusting sweeteners found in nature, or trusting artificial ones that are heavily influenced by corporate greed, it would seem considerably more prudent to use the natural ones.

Caveat Emptor
(Let the Buyer Beware)

Every day you are deluged with food-industry messages urging you to buy their products—from the sophisticated fake third-party "science" aimed at adults to colorful cartoon characters shilling to children. It's important to remember that their goal is to sell you the greatest number of items they can, for the highest price possible, made at the lowest achievable cost. Nutrition, health, and safety are at best considered only in light of their potential adverse publicity or lawsuits.

Whenever you hear information about nutrition, food safety, or food-related legislation, always remember to be sensitive to the source of the information and ask:

- Who pays them?
- Who benefits?

If it turns out that they are associated with the manufacturers of the products they are praising, it would be wise to investigate further before believing what they say, especially if it involves using substances that could potentially end your life prematurely.

The FDA, on the other hand, is presumed to play a vital role in protecting you from unsafe drugs and food. The United States desperately requires an effective regulatory agency that can truly protect the public, as they did in the days of thalidomide. By allowing the corporations that market chemicals in the form of pharmaceutical drugs, food additives, pesticides, preservatives, coloring agents, and artificial sweeteners to financially support the FDA, our country has abandoned any hope for unbiased regulation and safety.

If the FDA cannot maintain its objectivity and honestly evaluate these issues, the health and safety of all Americans are at risk. Many corporations would have you believe it is absolutely harmless to consume their artificial and genetically modified products. The safety of artificial sweeteners and any other new products you use must be fully and independently investigated before you can believe they are absolutely safe. And these investigations must be free of any corporate conflict of interests.

There is a long history of synthetic products sold in the United States under the guise of improving health. To this day, the majority of people believe the myth that margarine is healthier than real butter despite the recent evidence that completely disputes this. The reality is, margarine is a hydrogenated oil, and those that consume hydrogenated oils have a significantly increased chance of heart disease over those who don't (and just eat real butter instead).[28, 29]

On a similar note, a large number of important, unanswered questions still remain about the long-term safety of artificial sweeteners. I believe your interests are best served by becoming better informed and developing a healthy dose of skepticism about these unnatural products. I also believe that there is compelling data to convince you that you simply cannot rely on the biased reviews of the FDA and industrial manufacturers to assure your safety.

But you can trust Mother Nature.

CHAPTER 7:
SWEET TRUTH

AN INTERVIEW WITH A
WHISTLE-BLOWING FDA PHYSICIAN

Dr. David Graham is the whistle-blowing FDA physician who testified before the Senate, in the wake of the Vioxx catastrophe, about the critical flaws in the FDA. Dr. Graham, in my opinion, is one of the leading health advocates in the United States and has suffered many personal challenges, as you will read, for standing up to the drug companies' assault on the American public.

His amazing story illustrates the fundamental flaws in the current structure of the FDA, and how it is virtually impossible for the FDA to protect you from the ravages of corporate greed. This is one of the most amazing interviews in health I have ever read, and it provides deep insights into why the system has gone so terribly wrong.

Dr. Graham gave this interview in early 2005 to Manette Loudon, who is the lead investigator and director of operations for Dr. Gary Null. It was published in the July 2005 issue of the Crusador *newspaper available at www.HealthLiesExposed.com. Reprinted with permission.[1]*

CRUSADOR: Dr. Graham, it's truly a pleasure to have the opportunity to interview you. Let me begin by asking you how long you've been with the FDA and what your current position is?

DR. GRAHAM: I've been with the FDA for 20 years. I'm currently the Associate Director for Science and Medicine in the Office of Drug Safety. That's my official job. But when I'm here today I'm speaking in my private capacity on my own time, and I do not represent the FDA. We can be pretty certain that the FDA would not agree with most of what I have to say. So with those disclaimers you know everything is okay.

CRUSADOR: On the November 23, 2004 PBS Online News Hour Program you were quoted as making the following statement: "I would argue that the FDA as currently configured is incapable of protecting America against another Vioxx. Simply put, FDA and the Center for Drug Evaluation Research (CDER) are broken." Since you've made that statement, has anything changed within the FDA to fix what's broken and, if not, how serious is the problem that we're dealing with here?

DR. GRAHAM: Since November, when I appeared before the Senate Finance Committee and announced to the world that the FDA was incapable of protecting America from unsafe drugs or from another Vioxx, very little has changed on the surface and substantively nothing has changed. The structural problems that exist within the FDA, where the people who approve the drugs are also the ones who oversee the post-marketing regulation of the drug, remain unchanged.

The people who approve a drug when they see that there is a safety problem with it are very reluctant to do anything about it because it will reflect badly on them. They continue to let the damage occur. America is just as at risk now as it was in November, as it was two years ago, and as it was five years ago.

CRUSADOR: In that same PBS program, you were also quoted saying, "The organizational structure within the CDER is currently geared towards the review and approval of new drugs. When a serious safety issue arises at post-marketing, the immediate reaction is almost always one of denial, rejection, and heat. They approved the drugs, so there can't possibly be anything wrong with it. This is an inherent conflict of interest." Based on what you're saying it appears that the FDA is responsible for protecting the interests of pharmaceutical companies and not the American people. Do you believe the FDA can protect the public from dangerous drugs?

DR. GRAHAM: As currently configured, the FDA is not able to adequately protect the American public. It's more interested in protecting the interests of industry. It views industry as its client, and the client is someone whose interest you represent. Unfortunately, that is the way the FDA is currently structured. Within the Center for Drug Evaluation and Research about 80 percent of the resources are geared towards the approval of new drugs and 20 percent is for everything else. Drug safety is about 5 percent.

The "gorilla in the living room" is new drugs and approval. Congress has not only created that structure, they have also worsened that structure through the PDUFA, the Prescription Drug User Fee Act, by which drug companies pay money to the FDA so they will review and approve its drug. So you have that conflict as well.

CRUSADOR: When did that go into effect?

DR. GRAHAM: The Prescription Drug User Fee Act came into play in 1992. It was passed by Congress as a way of providing the FDA with more funds so that it could hire more physicians and other scientists to review drug applications so that drugs would be approved more quickly. For industry, every day a drug is held up from being marketed, represents a loss of one to two million dollars of profit. The incentive is to review and approve the drugs as quickly as possible, and not stand in the way of profit-making. The FDA cooperates with that mandate.

CRUSADOR: And what about those new drugs? Are they any better than what already exists on the market?

DR. GRAHAM: It's a myth that is promulgated not only by industry but also by the FDA itself. It's a misperception that our lawmakers in Congress have as well and they've been fed this line by industry. Industry is saying there are all these lifesaving drugs that the FDA is slow to approve and people are dying in the streets because of it. The fact is that probably about two-thirds to three-quarters of the drugs that the FDA reviews are already on the market and are being reviewed for another indication.

So, for example, if I've got a drug that can treat bronchitis and now it's going to be used to treat a urinary tract infection, well, that's a new indication. But it's the same drug and we already know about the safety of the drug. There is nothing lifesaving there. There is nothing new. There is nothing innovative. A very small proportion of drugs represent a new drug that hasn't been marketed before. Most of those drugs are no better than the ones that exist. If you want to talk about breakthrough drugs—the ones that really make a difference in patients' lives and represent a revolution in pharmacology—we're talking about maybe one or two drugs a year. Most of them aren't breakthroughs and most of them aren't lifesaving, but they get treated as if they were.

CRUSADOR: Are you at liberty to discuss some of the problems your colleagues are finding with other drugs and if so, how widespread is the problem?

DR. GRAHAM: I'm really not at liberty to talk about things that pertain to my official duties at the FDA. I can talk in my private capacity, but I can't talk about material that would be confidential. What I can say is that there are a number of other scientists within the FDA who have also worked with drugs that they know are not safe, even though the FDA has approved or allowed them to remain on the market. They face some of the same difficulties that I do. The difference is that either the problem isn't as serious in terms of the numbers of people that were injured or that it's a fatal reaction—they're not willing to expose themselves to retaliation by the FDA—and retaliation would surely follow.

CRUSADOR: Do you think we should have any confidence in the FDA and, if so, can you elaborate on what they do that you feel benefits the American people?

DR. GRAHAM: In terms of confidence in what the FDA does, there are two things that the FDA determines when it looks at a drug: it determines whether or not a drug is safe and it determines whether or not it's effective. Regarding the determination of drug effectiveness, I think the FDA does a pretty good job. If the FDA says that the drug will have a particular effect, probably for many of the patients who take the drug it will actually have that effect. If the FDA says a given drug will lower blood pressure and you're somebody who has high blood pressure, there's a good chance that the drug will have an effect that lowers your blood pressure. That has to do with the rigor with which they force the drug companies to establish that the drug actually has an effect.

On the safety side, I think that the American public can't be very confident. They can have some confidence because it turns out that most drugs are remarkably safe. But, when there are unsafe drugs, the FDA is very likely to err on the side of industry. Rarely will they keep a drug from being marketed or pull a drug off the market. A lot of this has to do with the standards that the FDA uses for safety. When they look at efficacy, they assume that the drug doesn't work and the company has to prove that the drug does work. When they look at safety it's entirely the opposite.

The FDA assumes the drug is safe and now it's up to the company to prove that the drug isn't safe. Well, that's a no-brainer. What company on earth is going to try to prove that the drug isn't safe? There's no incentive for the companies to do things right. The clinical trials that are done are too small, and as a result it's very unusual to find a serious safety problem in these clinical trials. Safety flaws are discovered after the drug gets on the market.

CRUSADOR: I read somewhere that a drug only has to be better than a sugar pill.

DR. GRAHAM: Right. The standard that the FDA uses to approve a drug is primarily "does the drug work?" That's what they call efficacy. Most often, they'll compare the drug against something called a placebo or a sugar pill. It's basically something that doesn't have a medical effect. The assumption is that the drug will be no different than the sugar pill. The FDA puts the onus on the drug company to conduct a clinical trial to show that the drug is different from a sugar pill. The way the FDA's approval standards are, the drug does not necessarily have to have a very great effect in order to be approved. The drug might lower your blood pressure by just a few millimeters of mercury, but the FDA will say we can approve it because it *does* lower your blood pressure.

Now, would that be a benefit or are there other drugs out there—many other drugs—that patients could take instead that would lower their blood pressure by ten or fifteen or twenty millimeters? The FDA doesn't really care about that. What happens is the drug gets marketed. You've got two drugs that are out there— one drug that effectively lowers your blood pressure a substantial degree and another drug that barely lowers your blood pressure at all. The company that has that second drug markets it like it's this breakthrough medicine. It lowers your blood pressure and they have all these glitzy ads, direct-to-consumer advertising.

Lots of patients and lots of doctors will use that medication. What happens in the process is these patients are actually in a sense being denied a more effective treatment because the FDA doesn't require that drugs that come on to market be at least equivalent to, or better than, the drugs that are already there. All they have to do is be better than a sugar pill.

CRUSADOR: When you consider the financial impact your whistle blowing has had on the pharmaceutical industry do you have any fears that your life may be in jeopardy?

DR. GRAHAM: I have tried not to think about that. In the work that I've done, I've never really thought about what the financial impact would be on any particular company. I put that out of my mind because my primary concern is whether or not the drug is safe. If it's not safe, how unsafe is it and how many people are being hurt by it? In terms of when I identify an unsafe drug, to me it doesn't really matter what drug company it is. I've helped to get ten different drugs off the market, and they're from ten different drug companies. It's not a vendetta against any particular drug company. I have to hope that the drug companies don't take it personally. I'm just a scientist doing my job, and I have to leave the rest to God to protect me.

CRUSADOR: Has anyone tried to silence you and stop you from becoming a whistleblower?

DR. GRAHAM: Prior to my Senate testimony in mid-November of 2004, there was an orchestrated campaign by senior level FDA managers to intimidate me so that I would not testify before Congress. This intimidation took several forms. One attack came from our acting center director who contacted the editor of *The Lancet*, the prestigious medical journal in the United Kingdom, and intimated to the editor that I had committed scientific misconduct and that they shouldn't publish a paper that I had written showing that Vioxx increases the risks of heart attack. This high-level FDA official never talked to me about this allegation. He just went directly to *The Lancet*.

The second attack was from other high-level FDA officials who contacted Senator Grassley's office and attempted to prevent Senator Grassley and his staff from supporting me and calling me as a witness. They knew that if they could disarm Senator Grassley that would neutralize me.

The third attack came from senior FDA officials who contacted Tom Devine, my attorney at the Government Accountability Project, and attempted to convince him that he should not represent me because I was guilty of scientific misconduct; I was a bully, a demigod and a terrible person that couldn't be trusted. These people were posing as whistleblowers themselves ratting on another whistleblower. Some of these senior level FDA officials were in my supervisory chain and are people I work for. They were involved in a coordinated attempt to discredit me and to smear my name and to prevent me from giving testimony.

There's one other thing that happened the week before I testified. The Acting Commissioner of the FDA invited me to his office and offered me a job in the commissioner's office to oversee the revitalization of drug safety for the FDA if I would just leave the Office of Drug Safety and come to the commissioner's office. Obviously he had been tipped off by people in the Senate Finance Committee who are sympathetic to the FDA's status quo that I was going to be called as a witness. To preempt that, he offers me this job, which basically would have been exile to a fancy title with no real ability to have an impact. This was a conspiracy and it was coordinated and there was collaboration among senior level FDA officials. What a mess!

CRUSADOR: All of these attacks backfired on them. Tell us a little bit about that.

DR. GRAHAM: Well, Senator Grassley and his staff quickly realized that what they were saying about me was fabricated. The editor of *The Lancet* also realized that what the high-level FDA officials were saying to him was a pack of lies. He sent e-mails to them saying it looked to him as if they were trying to interfere with his editorial process. He was very savvy to what these people were doing. Tom Devine, as he said publicly, was very interested in doing the right thing. He said, "We don't want to protect somebody who's a law-breaker and who really isn't representing the truth so produce your evidence." They had no evidence because there is no evidence. But I produced my evidence. I showed him all the documentation, all the e-mails, and the reports that I've written. They flunked every test and I passed every test.

In all of the criticism I have received relating to Vioxx and drug safety, they've never attacked the work or the science that I've done or the results that I've come to. What they've done is call me names. The ad hominem attack is the last refuge of the indefensible. They don't have an argument that's substantial. They know that they're vulnerable. They know that they've disserved the American people. The FDA is responsible for 140,000 heart attacks and 60,000 dead Americans. That's as many people as were killed in the Vietnam

War. Yet the FDA points the finger at me and says, "Well, this guy's a rat, you can't trust him," but nobody is calling them to account. Congress isn't calling them to account. For the American people, it's dropped off the radar screen. They should be screaming because this can happen again.

CRUSADOR: On CNN with Lou Dobbs you said that there was a certain "culture" that exists at the FDA. Can you explain what you meant by that?

DR. GRAHAM: The FDA has a very peculiar culture. It runs like the army so it's very hierarchal. You have to go through the chain of command, and if somebody up above you says that they want things done in a particular way, well, they want it done in a particular way. The culture also views industry as the client.

They're serving industry rather than the public. In fact, when a former office director for the Office of Drug Safety criticized me and tried to get me to change a report I'd written on another drug—Arava—he said to me and to a colleague who was a co-author on this report that "industry is our client." I begged to differ with him. I said, "No, industry is not the client, it's the American people, the people who pay our taxes. That's who we're here to serve." He said, "No! Industry is our client." I ended the conversation by saying, "Well, industry may be your client, but it will never be my client."

Another aspect to the culture at the FDA is that it overvalues the benefits of drugs and undervalues the risks of drugs. And so the FDA will always say to you, "Well, we're leaving this drug on the market because the benefits exceed the risks." Well, the FDA has never assessed the benefit of any drug that it's ever approved. It works on what's called efficacy. Does the drug work or not? Does it lower your blood pressure or does it lower your blood sugar? Not: Does it prolong your life? Does it prevent you from having a heart attack? Those are benefits. All they focus on is efficacy.

For example, ask the FDA why on earth they didn't ban high-dose Vioxx after the VIGOR Study showed in early 2000 that it increased the risk of heart attack by 500 percent. High-dose Vioxx was approved for the short-term treatment of acute pain. What earthly benefit was there that exceeds a 500 percent increase in heart attack risk? Ask the FDA to produce its benefit analysis that shows that the benefits exceed the risks. It doesn't exist. The FDA has never looked at benefit. The FDA just says to the American people, "The benefits exceed the risks. Trust me. Believe me." If you held the FDA to its proof the American people would see how badly served they've been by the FDA and its culture that belittles safety in the drug companies' interest.

If the FDA were to pull a drug due to safety issues, it would hurt the marketing of the drug. It might also call into question why they approved the drug in the first place. Therefore, you get this culture of cover-up, this culture of suppression, this culture of denial, and this culture that demonstrates above all else that industry is the client and not the American people.

CRUSADOR: Have your peers turned against you?

DR. GRAHAM: No. I've been very fortunate. Tom Devine at GAP [Government Accountability Project] has told me that the experience of a typical whistleblower is that they'll have the support of their peers, but the peers will be so afraid of retaliation that they won't express that support in public.

I've had a very different experience. I've been basically embraced by my peers as someone who has said what they want to say and what they wished they had been able to say and that they recognize as the truth. They're really proud of the fact that I've said it and they're not afraid to be seen with me. They're not afraid to work with me. I've been pretty fortunate in that way.

Now with management it's been another story. Upper management avoids me and doesn't talk to me. I could be walking down the hall and I'll say hello, and they'll act like I'm not there. They don't give me interesting work assignments. They don't call me in to consult on things that I should be consulted on even though I am the senior epidemiologist in the Office of Drug Safety with more experience than any of the other people there. I'm looked up to by the scientific staff because of that expertise. Basically, I feel like I'm in the Gulag [prison].

CRUSADOR: How do you cope with that going to work each day?

DR. GRAHAM: It's difficult. It's a mind game. They're hoping that I'll just become very frustrated and disillusioned and leave or that I'll slip up in some way so that they can take some sort of action against me. As Tom Devine at GAP has said, I have to be "Saint David." I can't afford to make any mistakes. That's very difficult and it is a little bit discouraging. But I've been a target of retaliation in the past. You take ten drugs off the market—well, no good deed goes unpunished at the FDA. I've experienced retaliation with many of those other episodes but not as severe as what I've experienced with Vioxx. This is the first time that my job was actually in jeopardy and where the FDA actually intended to fire me. That was stopped only because Senator Grassley intervened. He put the heat on the FDA and told them, "Lay off. This guy has told the truth. He's helped America. Whose side are you on?"

CRUSADOR: Were there any warnings that Vioxx was a problem? Did you see the disaster coming?

DR. GRAHAM: I think that I was afraid that there would be a disaster, but I only became aware of this with the publication of the VIGOR Study, which was this large clinical trial that was done that showed that Vioxx increased the risk of heart attack fivefold. That study was published in November of 2000. It was written, performed, and paid for by industry. What industry concluded was not that Vioxx increases the risks of heart attack, but that the drug they were comparing it against—Naproxen—decreased the risk of heart attack. I knew that was not a sustainable argument. There was no way that Naproxen was that protective against heart attacks. Clearly, Vioxx was the problem. I knew that Vioxx was on the road to becoming a blockbuster drug (twenty million users). All the ingredients were there for a disaster.

The FDA is responsible in so far as it could have prevented much of the damage, heart attacks, and deaths simply by banning the high-dose Vioxx back in mid-2000 when they knew the results of the VIGOR Study. But the FDA did nothing for almost two years. They were "negotiating" with the company over a label. What did the label accomplish? Nothing! Before the label 17 or 18 percent of people who took Vioxx took the high dose. After the label change 17 or 18 percent were still taking the high dose. High-dose use didn't change at all.

People didn't read the label, and if they read the label they wouldn't know what to do anyway because it was very confusing. The right thing to do would have been to pull the high dose off the market because there is no benefit for short-term relief of acute pain that exceeds this risk. The FDA made bad decisions based on its culture and its institutionalized biases that favor industry, and, as a result, thousands of Americans died. Americans and Congress should be screaming bloody murder. They should be beating on the doors of the FDA demanding change.

CRUSADOR: It's estimated that over two hundred thousand people a year die from prescription drugs. Do you see this as a serious problem and do you think many of these treatments are more dangerous than the disease itself?

DR. GRAHAM: Death from adverse drug reactions is one of the leading causes of death in the United States. It turns out that most of these adverse reactions are actually what are expected in the sense that they are an extension of the drug's action. For example, we know that drugs for diabetes can lower your blood sugar. If you're more sensitive to the drug than the normal person and it lowers your blood sugar too much, causing you to have a seizure while driving your car and you get killed, well, you died from an adverse drug reaction, but it wasn't something unexpected.

The blood thinner Coumadin is another example. That drug provides a benefit, but it is also responsible for probably more deaths than any single drug currently marketed. But it has a recognized benefit and there aren't other drugs to do what it does or to do what it does well. So physicians accept that there are patients who are in a serious situation and who might die without the drug, so they take it.

Yes, drugs cause a lot of harm. Unfortunately, we haven't quantified the benefits. For most of these drugs it's more belief. It's faith. We have faith that they'll confer a benefit, but the FDA hasn't demonstrated that they confer a benefit. We're getting much better at quantitating the risks. In the future, what we need to do is just take the risks and look hard and dispassionately at what the real benefits are. If the benefits aren't there, we shouldn't be having discussions about labeling the drug. You need to weed the garden patch of drugs that aren't doing what they're supposed to do. The FDA has not been very good about that. It likes to cultivate all these weeds.

CRUSADOR: In a perfect world, what role do you see the FDA playing in our nation's health?

DR. GRAHAM: In a perfect world, I think the FDA would need to be restructured. If it were restructured properly, I think that it could actually provide a great benefit to the public health. I would recommend several changes. First, I would separate safety and post-marketing from the pre-marketing. I would create a separate center for product safety. Actually, Senators Grassley and Dodd have recently introduced legislation to create an independent center for post-marketing safety that would serve to protect the American people from unsafe drugs. This isn't happening now.

On the pre-marketing side, the FDA needs to pay greater attention to safety. They need to have larger clinical trials. They need to compare drug products against other drugs that treat the same indication rather than comparing a drug against a sugar pill. What we want in the end are drugs that actually have better benefit.

The FDA also needs to determine the post-marketing benefits of a drug. I've done that for several drugs. How many people are actually benefiting? How many people are living longer versus those who are having their lives shortened? Only when you have that kind of information can you make rational decisions about a medication. The times when I've done the benefit analysis, I've been chastised, criticized, and suppressed by the FDA. These benefit analyses should be done as a matter of routine.

There is a lot that the FDA could do to improve, but the changes aren't going to happen on their own. Congress is going to have to make them happen. There's an expression, "The zebra doesn't change its stripes nor the leopard its spots." The FDA isn't going to change the way it does business. Changes will have to be imposed from outside.

CRUSADOR: How you do feel about direct-to-consumer advertising?

DR. GRAHAM: Direct-to-consumer advertising in general is a great disservice to the American people. We see wonderful ads of people demonstrating their health, whether they're skating across the ice or doing their tai chi. Madison Avenue knows that a picture is worth a thousand words, so they convey an image and a message, and it makes an impression on patients and on physicians. It creates needs or desires where there really isn't a need or a desire.

There was a recent study in *The Journal of the American Medical Association* that showed that if patients mentioned a drug that they've seen on television to their physician they were much more likely to be prescribed that drug by the doctor. Drug companies know this. That's why they do it. Would the Vioxx disaster have been as great and as large in the absence of direct-to-consumer advertising? I submit that the numbers would have been far lower than what they were. Direct-to-consumer advertising is part of what made Vioxx a blockbuster drug. It helped to rev the market up to get people to want to use the drug.

Clearly, direct-to-consumer advertising does not serve the American people well. Madison Avenue is smarter than the most intelligent American. That's why they make so much money and that's why the drug companies go to them to sell their products. We're not living in a neutral world where the information we're getting is objective and unbiased. It might be that the average American, given all the data, all the facts, and all the information in an objective way could make an intelligent, rational decision. But we don't live in that kind of world.

We live in a world where what we're seeing is a visual image of these people being vital and healthy and cured of their illnesses. And it's all because of this little pill that they're taking. A patient with that condition says, "I want to be just like that person." So they go to the doctor and say, "I want that pill." Are their lives changed? Maybe some people's lives are changed, but I think most aren't.

CRUSADOR: What do you think people hear when they're watching the ad and after the ad they list all the possible side effects?

DR. GRAHAM: I don't think it registers. You have the visual image that conveys one message. Then you have the voice that's speaking over this pictorial being shown telling you what this drug is good for. Then at the end the auctioneer gets on and says, "You know this drug could cause . . . ," and they rattle off twenty-five different things in three seconds. You're lucky if you hear anything. I don't think that people come away with it, and they certainly don't come away with any sense of how likely it is to happen because the visual image overpowers anything that gets said.

It's the same with the ads that appear in magazines. Companies are required to put some of the labeling in the ad. You have the ad on the one side—that's the picture. It shows this person being healthy because they take this pill. The fine print is all on the next page. People aren't going to read the fine print. It's the same thing with labeling for physicians. Physicians don't read product labels. Where do they learn about drugs? They learn about drugs from the detail person from the drug company or from other colleagues who have used the drug. They're not learning it from the labeling.

CRUSADOR: Do you think there is a criminal cover-up going on between the FDA and Big Pharma to approve dangerous drugs that sicken and kill Americans?

DR. GRAHAM: I have no knowledge of criminal activity and I'm sure there are legal standards for what's criminal and what's not. I do think that there is an institutional bias at the FDA that says we will look for a way to say "yes" to the approval of any drug that comes down the pipe. If a drug is so bad that they can't find a reason to approve it, they won't. But, if there is any way that they can approve the drug, they will. The way this is done is by what's called the "indication."

Why is it that you're going to take the drug? Maybe you're going to take it because you have high blood pressure. Maybe you'll take it because you have high cholesterol. That's the indication. A company may come in with a drug and want to get it approved for five different indications. One of them is a really insignificant indication that affects a very small number of people. The main indication might affect millions of people. The drug doesn't show efficacy for that major indication, but they're able to somehow or another approve the small indication.

So the drug gets approved for this narrow indication, but the FDA and the drug company both know that it's going to be used for that other indication. It's going to be used "off-label." Then, the FDA turns around and says that they don't regulate the "off-label" use of drugs. No. But they aid and abet it. They allow it to happen and, in many instances, "off-label" use of a drug product is a public health threat. The FDA has a responsibility to protect the public health. The FDA should be intervening, but they don't. In my own experience I have seen multiple examples where I've heard people say, "We can't ask a company to put that in the labeling because the company will say no." Or, "We can't do that because that will decrease their marketing. We've got to try to approve this drug. Let's see if we can give them this small indication. At least it's giving them something. You've got to find a way to say yes."

That is the typical attitude of the FDA culture. I think Congress is partially responsible for that because when they issued the PDUFA, the Prescription Drug User Fee Act, what they were really saying was, "We want you to review these drug applications more quickly because you're keeping lifesaving medicines from the American people." That's the line they were fed by Big Pharma. So they pressure the FDA, and the FDA gets the message. It's a really pernicious system. I think it's unfortunate. There are many people from the FDA who have examples that they unfortunately can't talk about. They'd lose their job and maybe get thrown in prison because you can't discuss confidential and trade secret information. But the fact is, these things happen at the FDA, and there have been multiple examples in the past where one could see evidence of that.

CRUSADOR: Did your faith as a devout Roman Catholic play any role in the decisions you made to put your career on the line to report the truth?

DR. GRAHAM: It did in so far as my faith forms my conscience. It's sort of my sense of what's right and what's wrong and what I am and am not responsible for. I was in a situation here with Vioxx where I was invited by Senator Grassley's office to testify. I could have told them no, but then they would have subpoenaed me. So of course I went peaceably. I was faced with this dilemma. Should I lay it on the line and tell them the way it really is, or do I kind of downplay it? There are ways of doing that.

What I concluded was that I'm now being given the opportunity to tell the truth to the people who are in a position to actually make a difference. I can't make a difference. I can't change the FDA, but Congress can. If I don't tell them the truth, then I'm now responsible, in part, for future deaths. I don't want to become a co-conspirator with the FDA in what happens with Vioxx because tens of thousands of people were injured or killed because of the FDA's disregard for safety. If I keep quiet about that, now I'm part of the problem. I'm one of them, and, at that point, then my conscience asks me, "You know what the truth is. Are you going to speak it or aren't you?"

So I went ahead and did that and prayed that it all works out well for me personally. That I have a job and I'll be able to support my family, that I'm protected from retaliation, that maybe some good will come out of that. My faith plays a role, but it wasn't a direct teaching of the church. You have to do x, y, and z, but it's the faith as I've internalized it. My conscience is formed by the voice of Christ speaking internally to me. That's what the conscience is: it's the voice of God speaking to each and every one of us about what's right and what's wrong. I knew what was right. If I walked away from that, nobody else would have to do anything. I'd be beating myself up because my conscience would condemn me. So, yes, faith plays a part in everything that I do. It's not saying I'm a saint, because I'm not. But I can't separate who I am from my religious faith. It's all part of the same person.

CRUSADOR: Do you think Congress genuinely wants to fix the problems at the FDA or are too many politicians influenced by the pharmaceutical industry?

DR. GRAHAM: I don't know what Congress will do in the end. My hope is that they will act decisively to reform the FDA and make the American people safer by having strong post-marketing. Will that happen or not? I don't know. I think there are many people in Congress who see this as a serious problem and who very much want to see a change. I think, at the same time, there are other people who don't think it's such a bad problem, and many of those people honestly believe that. For those people, I'd say they haven't seen the evidence so they don't really understand how bad the problem is. There are undoubtedly some people who are influenced by industry. Does that influence their judgment in the end? I don't know.

They'd probably say no, it doesn't. Maybe at a conscious level it doesn't. But we have the same phenomenon in the scientific world where we look at research studies that are funded by industry and studies that are funded by government, by National Institutes of Health or the Medical Research Council in the United Kingdom. Multiple studies have been done that have shown that if your study is funded by industry you are much likelier—about five times more likely—to come up with the result that's favorable to the drug company than if your study on the same subject is funded by an independent body unrelated to the company.

Now, are the researchers who did this study biased? Are they consciously cheating and manipulating the data and everything else? No. I don't think that's happening at all, but the fact is if the study is funded by industry it's much more likely to be favorable to industry. Without attributing bad motivations to the scientists doing those studies, all I can do is point to a strong correlation.

With Congress I would be concerned that there could be a strong correlation there because Pharma is very bright. They fund as many politicians as they can. They get to the Republicans and the Democrats. Look at the funding on the major committees: the Health, Education, Labor and Pension Committee in the Senate or the Oversight and Investigations Subcommittee in the House. *The Wall Street Journal* reported recently that many people on these committees are funded by industry to a substantial degree. Industry knows how to exercise influence. What we have to do is overcome that influence with evidence, and then rely on the fact that, at the end of the day, the Congress will do what's best for the American people.

Will that happen? I don't know because then it gets embroiled in politics. You know, Republicans versus Democrats, the left versus the right, conservatives versus liberals. Yet, what we're talking about is public health and public health is nonpartisan. I can say this with certainty. For every member of the House of Representatives, somebody in their district died because of Vioxx. Somebody in their district had a heart attack because of Vioxx. For every Senator in the Senate, many more people in their state died because of Vioxx or had a heart attack because of Vioxx. It doesn't matter whether it's a red state or a blue state. Those are human beings and what we're talking about is public health. What I'm hoping is that Congress will respond. There is a problem and the evidence is overwhelming, but we'll just have to wait and see.

CRUSADOR: What are your thoughts on President Bush's attempt to pass tort reform, which would protect most pharmaceutical companies from lawsuits except in the most egregious cases?

DR. GRAHAM: I think it's dangerous and wrong for the following reasons. We already have an FDA that's been neutralized by industry and sees industry as its client. The Center for Drug Evaluation and the Office of New Drugs dominates drug safety so that the drug safety is not independent. Drug safety can't protect the American people. So government now isn't going to protect the average citizen from the consequences of unsafe drugs. The only alternative they have left is the legal system—the tort system. It's not a wonderful system. It would be much better if we had effective post-marketing regulation so that we could get bad drugs off the market before they hurt more people, but that's been neutralized. All that's left to people now is the courts. That's the only way we have of getting companies to change their behavior.

What tort reform will do is remove that threat as well. It's basically giving companies immunity because now the people who are injured by the drugs can't recover damages that might actually mean something to industry. I mean, $250,000 for damages . . . they blow that in one ad campaign. To them that's nothing. But a lawsuit for multiple millions of dollars has more of an impact. Now, is that optimal? No. But the fact is that since we have a regulatory agency that doesn't regulate and we have a public health agency that doesn't protect the public, we have thousands of people who are being injured by products that the FDA knows are unsafe. The FDA knew there was a problem with Vioxx. They knew it was a big problem back in mid-2000 yet did nothing about it.

There has to be a system in place that reins companies in. If the FDA isn't going to exercise control over companies, then who will? How will it happen? I don't think that working through the courts and lawsuits is a particularly effective way of doing it; but it's the only recourse we have now, and that will be removed as well. You can demonize the trial lawyers but I think that there are patients who are severely injured by drugs. The defense is, "It's on the labels so we're protected." The problem is that nobody reads the labels so how do they protect anyone? The FDA should be making those decisions.

CRUSADOR: What can you tell us about all the antidepressants on the market that millions of children are taking?

DR. GRAHAM: In early 2004, SSRI antidepressants and suicidal behavior was a big safety issue. The FDA had suppressed a report written by a colleague of mine in drug safety and had prevented him from presenting this information in an advisory committee meeting. That information leaked to the media, embarrassing the FDA because it had been caught suppressing very important information—that most of the antidepressants don't work for treating children. Someone in my supervisory chain initiated a criminal investigation to identify the person who had leaked this information to the media. It turns out that the investigation ordered by these FDA officials was illegal. They broke federal laws—at least two or three federal laws—in ordering this investigation.

I think it's well established that depression is very common in adolescence. With the antidepressants that we have on the market right now only one of them has been shown to work in children, Fluoxetine or Prozac. All the other SSRI antidepressants are no better than sugar pills. However, if you were to read the labeling for these drugs it doesn't point that fact out, so patients think one SSRI is as good as another. This is another way that the FDA has betrayed the American public and has betrayed the public health.

With the SSRI and antidepressants, what the FDA should have insisted on was a signed informed consent at the time a child was going to be treated. That informed consent would say three things. One, these are the antidepressants that are available. Only Fluoxetine has been shown to work for depression in children. All the other drugs are no better than placebos. That's point two. No better than placebos. No better than sugar pills. Third, all of these drugs appear to have the ability to increase the risk of suicidal behavior. As a parent, if I see that in writing and the psychiatrist or GP is going to write the prescription and put my child on some drug other than Fluoxetine, I can say, "Doc, why are you putting my child on a drug that doesn't work in kids?"

The FDA didn't want patients to have that information so they refused to have signed informed consent. The companies didn't want the patients to have that information because all of a sudden the "off-label" use of these drugs would dry up. So whose interest was being served there?

CRUSADOR: How do you feel about taking the approval process out of the hands of the FDA?

DR. GRAHAM: Well, where would you put it? If you put it somewhere else, they're going to eventually become co-opted the way the FDA has been co-opted. I think the most that we could probably hope for is to try to disassociate the industry pressures from the approval decision. You have to change the culture of the organization, and you have to change the incentives in the organization. The culture and the incentives that the FDA operates by would have to be changed, and Congress can do that through legislation and by establishing different standards for how a drug gets approved. Not only do you have to show that the drug is effective, but you've got to show that it works as well or better than other drugs that treat that indication. You've got to prove to me that the drug is safe, not that the drug is harmful because you're never going to prove to me that the drug is harmful. You set up stringent standards of evidence that might lead to the approval of safe drugs that actually have benefits to the population.

Then pair that up with an independent post-marketing regulation. Currently, the pre-market people who approve the drug decide what happens after it's on the market. If the drug needs to come off the market, they're the ones who have to say yes at the end of the day. The people at the FDA who approved the drug, the Office of New Drugs, they are the single greatest obstacle when it comes to removing unsafe drugs from the market. I can vouch for that from personal experience. What you have to do is you have to take that responsibility and power away from them and put it with the group who sees their mission as serving the public and protecting the public health from unsafe drugs. I think if you do those two things you'd be a long way towards getting the FDA on the right footing.

Also, it would probably be beneficial not to have the FDA's funding come from industry. He who pays the piper calls the tune, and we now have a captured agency. Industry underwrites more than 50 percent of the Center for Drug Evaluation's budget. When industry yanks the chain, whose neck is going to get tugged? The Center for Drug Evaluation! If industry isn't happy with them and the funding dries up what are we going to do? We're going to have to let half our people go. The program is going to shrink. Congress is going to be jumping up and down on our back. So it's a captured agency and America is not well served when industry is calling all the shots. Yes, industry has a right to make a legitimate profit from marketing products that help the American people. But you shouldn't have a situation that just basically leaves the American public defenseless. And that's what we have right now. We're virtually defenseless.

CRUSADOR: Are there other Vioxx's out there? Do you think this will repeat itself at this high-profile level?

DR. GRAHAM: At this current moment, I don't think there are other drugs out there that are as bad as Vioxx in terms of the enormous numbers of people that were hurt. During my Senate testimony I did mention that there were five other drugs that I thought the FDA really needed to reevaluate because, in my estimation, the benefit to risk was misjudged. After I named those five drugs the FDA was in the media saying that I did junk science and that these drugs were safe and effective and that I was a crackpot. However, recently the FDA announced that they were going to take Bextra off the market. Well, Bextra was one of the five I mentioned.

They announced that, with Acutane, they were going to impose a restricted distribution system. Well, I had recommended a restricted distribution system fifteen years ago. The major problem with Acutane is that it's just so widely overused that it causes an enormous amount of potential harm to pregnancy exposure. If we restricted the use of the drug to the small number of women who really need it each year, the problem would be pretty much resolved. But the FDA didn't want to do that because it would interfere with company profits. If you restrict the distribution and only one-tenth of the people who are getting it now are getting it tomorrow, profit will drop 90 percent. Of course, companies aren't going to go along with that and the FDA isn't going to do anything that's going to harm corporate profit.

After my Senate testimony, the FDA announced that they can look at other drugs—not only the other three of the five that I mentioned. There are other drugs on the market that I prefer not to talk about that the FDA knows are killing people. Ten or a hundred people a year are dying because of the use of a particular drug. Hundreds or maybe thousands of people are being hospitalized each year. For some of those drugs, the benefits do exceed the risks. For others, it's clear that more could and should be done and maybe that means restricting the distribution of the drug's use or maybe it means banning an indication for the drug saying the drug should not be used for particular indications. Maybe it would be something like with the SSRIs where I believe there should be signed informed consent so that parents will know that the drug the doctor is prescribing for their son or daughter actually doesn't work in children.

I think that there are many things that can be done that haven't been done. There are other unsafe drugs out there, and the nature of our business is that a drug could be approved tomorrow that turns out to be the next Vioxx and we won't know until it happens. Then the question is, how quickly do we identify the problem and how quickly do we take effective action against it? We're pretty good at identifying these problems quickly. Where the FDA falls flat on its face is that there is a long period of time in which it does nothing. Then what it normally does is woefully inadequate and ineffective and as a result the body count mounts and that needs to be changed. Maybe Congress will change that.

CRUSADOR: Let's talk about incentives. When you say incentives what do you mean? For example, working at the FDA, is their pay somehow based on how many drugs they approve?

DR. GRAHAM: Currently, the performance evaluations for managers at the FDA are built around the drug review. How many reviews did they get done? Did they meet their PDUFA deadlines? It looks bad if you miss your PDUFA deadlines. The unspoken mores—what's expected—is that you're going to approve as many of these drugs as you can. There has to be an overwhelming reason for you not to approve. Frequently what will happen is that these medical officers in their review will recommend that a drug not be approved and they get overruled by the higher-ups because the higher-ups are answering to a different set of incentives. You have to change that. A lot of that comes from the leaders. What I want to see is, does the drug really make a difference? Is it beneficial?

There are many classes of drugs where we've got ten or fifteen members of that class. They all lower your blood pressure. They all lower your cholesterol. Another one comes along and the FDA feels its obligation to approve it. Why? Maybe the standard should be that for the drugs that come later in a class, they've got to show that they're actually better than the drugs on the market because we've already got these other drugs that work. That would create incentives maybe within industry to develop drugs that are better than the ones that are already there. Currently, the way the incentives are for industry, it's safer to do a "me too" drug, another drug in the same class.

CRUSADOR: Do you think that the FDA should not be partially funded by industry?

DR. GRAHAM: I think that PDUFA funding for the FDA is a mistake.

CRUSADOR: Can you explain that a little more clearly because most people don't know what PDUFA funding is?

DR. GRAHAM: The drug companies pay a substantial amount of money to the FDA at the time that they bring a drug application for approval in order for the FDA to review the drug. Basically, it's a tax. It's a fee. Industry pays the fee, and the FDA will review the drug application. But the real expectation is from the company: "We've paid our money, now approve our drug." That's basically how the FDA reacts as well. I think that the funding for the FDA should be independent of the industry that it's regulating, and I think in the scientific field there's good evidence to support this notion. Industry money is influencing the decisions that get made, and it creates this incentive structure. You have this culture, you have these expectations, you have pressure from Congress. All of them come to a head at the FDA and all of those incentives are in the direction of "approve the drug." That's what happens so I believe that the FDA is unduly influenced by industry and that undue influence is in part the result of industry money funding the FDA operations.

CRUSADOR: Dr. Graham, thank you for your commitment to your convictions and for sharing insights that drove you to save many lives.

DR. GRAHAM: You're welcome. I hope I've helped.

CHAPTER EIGHT: SWEET CONFECTIONS

ALTERNATIVES TO TABLE SUGAR AND ARTIFICIAL SWEETENERS

I have already reviewed the harmful effects of table sugar and high-fructose corn syrup (HFCS) on your body in chapter 1. But there are many other kinds of caloric sweeteners on the market, and I regularly receive questions from patients and Mercola.com subscribers regarding their safety and nutritional factors.

OTHER SWEETENERS	
Stevia	Sucanat®
Raw Honey	Turbinado Sugar
Date Sugar	Agave Syrup
Barley Malt	FOS
Brown Rice Syrup	Fructose
Lo Han Kuo	Fruit Juice Concentrate
Maple Syrup	Sugar Alcohols
Molasses	Tagatose

It's important to understand that most of these caloric sweeteners are simple sugar carbs and will cause a rise in your blood sugar level; they lack the necessary fibers, fat, or protein to slow down the absorption of the sugar into your bloodstream. And elevated blood sugar levels over time can lead to insulin resistance, metabolic syndrome, obesity, and diabetes. Furthermore, these sweeteners are deficient in most essential micronutrients that are necessary to achieve good health.

Some sweeteners are far safer for you than others, while some are far more processed, and dangerous, than their counterparts. Learning about them will help you decide which sweeteners are best for you to use, if you choose to use sweeteners at all.

But I strongly recommend that you consider significantly reducing or simply eliminating all sweeteners from your diet. This may seem like an unachievable goal, but when you are eating the food that is appropriate for your unique biochemistry, sugar cravings tend to almost magically disappear.

The basic concept is based on a system called "metabolic typing," which I reviewed more thoroughly in my previous book, *Dr. Mercola's Total Health Program* or, just type "metabolic typing" in Google or the search engine at Mercola.com.

The Dangers of Caloric Sweeteners

Most of the sweeteners presented in this chapter are more natural and safe for you than any artificial sweeteners; however, I still recommend consuming them with strict moderation, especially if you struggle with health challenges like weight or insulin and leptin control. (Leptin is a hormone that is found predominantly in your fat cells, and it affects body weight by controlling feeding behavior, hunger, body temperature, and energy expenditure; repeated blood sugar spikes from sugar can make you leptin resistant, just as they can make you insulin resistant.)

Let's face it. Two-thirds of Americans are overweight, and many others suffer from insulin-resistance syndromes like diabetes, high blood pressure, high blood cholesterol, and cancer. If you struggle with any of these conditions you will benefit from limiting all forms of sweeteners, even some of the healthy ones, until you get these conditions under control. If you are at all interested in feeling as young as possible, you will be more likely to achieve this worthy goal if you limit your sugar intake.

Another point you will want to consider is that frequently eating any type of sweetener, natural or artificial, will start desensitizing your appreciation of sweetness. This will force you to use progressively larger amounts of a sweetener to achieve a similar sensation of "sweet."

Whatever beneficial qualities a particular food might have, if it adversely raises your blood sugar levels, the damage it will cause will most likely far outweigh any short-term benefits you obtain from eating the food. For many of us the question, "What is the best sweetener to use?" is similar to, "Which would you rather be hit in the head with, a baseball bat or a golf club?"

Stevia

The sweetener I receive the most questions about by far is stevia. I've already discussed it a bit in terms of its treatment by the FDA; now we'll take a closer look at the sweetener itself.

Stevia is derived from a South American herb by the name of Stevia rebaudiana Bertoni. It is quickly gaining popularity as a natural, low-carbohydrate alternative to artificial sweeteners.

If you have weight or blood sugar issues, stevia can be an acceptable alternative to other natural sweeteners. It has virtually no calories, has little or no effect on blood sugar levels, and researchers have concluded that it is safe for human consumption.[1-3] If you must use a sweetener, this is probably the safest to use as it the least processed and has the highest density of sweetness per calorie of carbohydrate.

Using Stevia

Stevia is estimated to be two to three hundred times sweeter than sugar, so a little will go a long way. In fact, just a pinch will provide the same sweetening power of a teaspoon of sugar. Stevia is a good option for salad dressings, and as a beverage sweetener. With the appropriate adjustments, it is even possible to bake with stevia, although its lack of bulk compared to sugar makes it a little harder to work with. You may find that some brands of stevia are bitterer than others. Using stevia may take a little practice, but there are many cookbooks to help you along the way. A popular one is *The Stevia Cookbook*, by Donna Gates and Dr. Ray Sahelian.

Health Benefits

The stevia plant has been used as a traditional remedy for diabetes and gum disease among the indigenous people of Paraguay and other South American countries for over fifteen hundred years. Stevia has also been used for centuries as a medicine to treat a variety of other ailments, including blood sugar problems. In fact, research studies have shown that stevia may decrease or stabilize blood sugar levels, help to prevent cavities, and may also be useful in the treatment of high blood pressure.[4-7]

Safety Concerns

Many countries, most notably Japan, use stevia as a sweetener. In fact, as I mentioned earlier, hundreds of tons of stevia extracts have been consumed annually in Japan for almost thirty years in a number of different foods and beverages, with no reported side effects. They even used it in their version of Diet Coke™. Since the 1970s, the Japanese have conducted extensive research on stevia, and have found it to be completely safe.[8,9]

Nonetheless, certain countries, primarily the United States, Canada, and the European Union (EU), have refused to certify its use as a sweetener. In the United States, the FDA has not given stevia GRAS status; it is banned in food products and beverages, and can only be sold as a "nutritional supplement." In Canada, stevia can only be sold as an herb. (Chapter 6 contains a more complete summary of the FDA's treatment of stevia and the corporate manipulation behind it.)

Stevia's safety is allegedly being questioned based on an insufficient number of studies demonstrating its safety, and a few studies that show some potential problems. The opinions of the American and Canadian governments and the EU remain steadfast, even in light of widespread safe use in other countries and numerous studies that have shown no signs of toxicity.[10-12] In fact, Dr. Daniel Mowrey, who holds a doctorate in phytopharmacology and has studied stevia extensively, recently had this to say about its safety:

More elaborate safety tests [than had been done previously] were performed by the Japanese during their evaluation of stevia as a possible sweetening agent. Few substances have ever yielded such consistently negative results in toxicity trials as have stevia. Almost every toxicity test imaginable has been performed on stevia extract (concentrate) or stevioside at one time or another. The results are always negative. No abnormalities in weight change, food intake, cell or membrane characteristics, enzyme and substrate utilization, or chromosome characteristics. No cancer, no birth defects, no acute and no chronic untoward effects. Nothing.[13]

I also interviewed a prominent pharmacologist and toxicologist for his take on stevia. He is a consultant to the food industry and therefore wishes to remain nameless. He said the following:

Stevia has been blackballed by the FDA in order to protect the artificial sweetener companies. I would not call stevia a completely natural sweetener, as it is highly processed and the quality varies widely depending on the manufacturer. However, in my professional opinion, it is completely safe.

Our review of the research into the stevia safety controversy has allowed us to conclude that it is a safe product, and we endorse its use as a natural sweetener and an alternative to both sugar and artificial sweeteners. Further information on the controversy surrounding the safety of stevia can be found at stevia.net and steviacanada.com.

Natural Caloric Sweeteners

Your body is designed to optimally perform with minimally processed whole foods. When you start down the road of regularly using prepackaged and artificial foods, you dramatically increase your risk for developing all sorts of chronic degenerative health conditions. The best sweeteners to use in general are the ones that are as minimally processed as possible, like raw honey and date sugar, as long they are used on a *very* limited basis.

Organic Raw Honey

People have been eating raw honey for thousands of years. It may cause fewer problems than other sweeteners for the majority of healthy individuals who are eating a wholesome diet and use it in moderation. However, I believe that even if you are fit and don't struggle with insulin and leptin challenges, it would probably be wise to limit your use of raw honey. Remember your Paleolithic ancestors probably ate no more than four pounds of total sugars a year, which would come out to one tablespoon per day if honey was your exclusive form of sweetener. Beware of low-cost honey, which typically is neither raw nor certified organic, and probably has high levels of high-fructose corn syrup (HFCS).

Using Raw Honey

To be considered raw, the honey must never have been heated over 117°F. If you heat honey, you will destroy some of its nutritional benefits, especially its naturally high level of healthy enzymes. These enzymes are catalysts for chemical reactions that occur in your body and are present in almost all raw foods.

Honey is approximately one and a half times as sweet as sugar, so in any recipe in which it is replacing sugar, you should reduce the amount needed by half.[14] Although it does not spoil, honey can crystallize over time. If this happens, you can simply place the jar in some warm water (less than 117°F) until the crystals disappear.

Health Benefits

Raw honey is believed to possess a number of health benefits. It has been shown to have antimicrobial qualities, and can even be an effective remedy against common food-borne pathogens like E. coli and S. aureus. In fact, studies show that not only can it kill harmful bacteria in your bowels, but it may actually promote the growth of beneficial ones. Honey's antimicrobial qualities also extend to your mouth; honey can destroy the bacteria that contribute to cavities and reduce the acidity of your mouth, which inhibits bacteria's ability to stick to your teeth.[15, 16] Honey is also an effective topical treatment for burns, ulcers, and other types of wounds or abrasions, and has been used for centuries as a medicine in this manner to achieve remarkable recoveries for persistently infected nonhealing wounds. In addition to its antibacterial properties it may facilitate natural bioelectrical currents that stimulate wound repair.[17]

Safety Concerns

Raw honey of any kind should be avoided by pregnant or nursing mothers, and infants up to one year old. Some sources also recommend that immunocompromised persons, seniors, and those who take statin drugs for their cholesterol should also avoid raw honey, as they may lack the ability to destroy the botulism spores that are rarely present in honey.

Only about one-third of the annual total honey production in North America is natural, raw, organic honey. Bees produce this by converting botanical material like sap, nectars, or pollen into honey. The remainder of the honey is a type referred to as baker's honey, which is made by force feeding the bees HFCS, or other sugars, under twenty-four-hour hive lighting that fools the bees into overproducing outside the natural bee production times of spring and summer. The resulting "honey" is only partially regurgitated, meaning some of it is converted to real honey while the remainder is HFCS. One way you can test to see if the honey is genuine (beyond reading the label) is that baker's honey will burn at 140°; real honey will not.

Another advantage of 100 percent certified organic honey is that it is harvested without the use of the potentially toxic chemicals widely used in conventional beekeeping to control disease and parasites.

Date Sugar

As its name implies, date sugar is made from dates, using a simple process in which the dates are dehydrated and then ground into a powder. Date sugar is 85 percent sucrose, but also contains a concentrated amount of minerals, plus some beta-carotene, B vitamins, and folic acid, as well as some fiber.

Using Date Sugar

Date sugar has some limitations, as it does not dissolve easily and you cannot bake with it. It does work well in some recipes, however, and it can also be lightly sprinkled on foods or used to sweeten a smoothie. In any recipe that doesn't require the sweetener to be dissolved, you may substitute equal amounts of date sugar for white sugar. Be sure to store date sugar in a cool, dry place.

Health Benefits

Hyperactive children with ADD are usually best served by avoiding all grains, sugars, and processed foods. However, some researchers have found that giving date sugar to hyperactive children may have some benefit, due to its high concentration of the amino acid tryptophan, which is known to have a gentle, calming effect.[18]

But remember that date sugar is still sugar, and you will want to limit its use as much as possible.

More Processed Sweeteners

The next few sweeteners I will discuss are more processed than raw honey and date sugar, and as such are less preferable. However, they are all still technically natural and safe to consume in limited quantities. All of them will, however, raise your blood sugar:

- Barley malt
- Brown rice syrup
- Lo Han Kuo
- Maple syrup
- Molasses
- Sucanat
- Turbinado sugar

Barley Malt

Barley malt is another type of natural sweetener with a fairly long history. It is made from the sprouted grains of barley and has been used for thousands of years, especially in Asia. A large portion of barley malt syrup is maltose, the disaccharide composed of two glucose molecules.[19]

Using Barley Malt Syrup

Because of its liquid consistency, barley malt is not as versatile as some sweeteners when it comes to cooking; however, it can still be used in a variety of recipes with good success. But be sure to refrigerate it when it's not being used; unlike most of the other sweeteners, barley malt syrup can spoil.

Barley malt syrup can typically be found in the sweetener section of most health food stores and is also available for order on the Internet. Unfortunately, the majority of barley malt syrup in the United States is really just HFCS fraudulently labeled as barley syrup. The FDA is doing little to correct the situation among suppliers, because they do not see HFCS as harmful. One way to test for real barley syrup is to heat it to 140°F. If it darkens or caramelizes, it is HFCS or a blend of the two.

Health Benefits

In concentrated form barley malt is quite high in fiber and can actually be used as a treatment for constipation. Even nonconcentrated barley malt extract has 11.3 grams of fiber per cup. It is especially useful for treating constipated infants because they love its sweet flavor. Barley malt can also be useful in treating irritable bowel syndrome and other gastrointestinal disorders benefited by increased fiber intake.[20-22]

Brown Rice Syrup

Brown rice syrup is a traditional Asian sweetener made by fermenting brown rice with chemical enzymes that break down the natural starch content, followed by centrifuging, filtering, and purifying it to a dextrose consistency. This processing strips the rice syrup of most of its nutrients. Brown rice syrup is mostly maltose, and about 50 percent of the sweetness of sugar, so it is still better than sucrose in terms of its effect on raising blood sugar levels.

Using Brown Rice Syrup

You can substitute brown rice syrup in almost any recipe that calls for sugar, honey, corn syrup, maple syrup, or molasses, but because of its high water content it is difficult to bake with. To substitute it for sugar in a recipe, use ¼ cups of brown rice syrup for each cup of sugar, while using ¼ of a cup less of another liquid called for in the recipe. Brown rice syrup should be stored in a cool, dry place.

Lo Han Kuo

Lo Han Kuo (also spelled Lo Han Guo) is the fruit of Momordica grosvenori, a plant in the cucumber, melon, squash, and gourd family that is cultivated in the mountains of southern China. Extracts of this fruit can be up to 250 times sweeter than sugar.[23] It has a very strong black licorice flavor.

Producers of Lo Han Kuo say that because of its intense sweetness, the amounts normally used are so small that they are not likely to have any appreciable effect on human physiology. Like stevia, Lo Han Kuo has a naturally sweet taste and contains no sugar or calories.[24] Lo Han Kuo is said to be a great sweetener choice for hypoglycemia and diabetes, as it helps to control food and sugar cravings. It is also possible to cook or bake with Lo Han Kuo.

Health Benefits

In Chinese medicine, Lo Han Kuo has been used for thousands of years to treat a variety of ailments. It is said to be helpful for skin problems, sore throats, coughs, purifying the blood, and regulating the digestive tract. It is also described as a cooling, calming, relaxing herb that balances excess heat in the body and reduces stress. Classic Chinese medical texts even say it promotes longevity. To date, there have been very few studies in the United States to substantiate all of the aforementioned claims, although the results of one study do suggest that it could be useful for certain skin problems.[25]

Safety Concerns

Lo Han Kuo has a long history of use, without any safety issues. It has been given GRAS status for use in beverages, but due to its licorice aftertaste when heated, it is not often used as a sweetener by itself. It can be found in powdered and liquid form. One advantage of Lo Han Kuo over stevia is that it is less processed.

Maple Syrup

Maple syrup is made from the sap of large maple trees. It is high in trace minerals and is minimally processed, except that it is highly concentrated. It is so concentrated, in fact, that it takes thirty-five to fifty gallons of crude sap to make one gallon of maple syrup.

There are four different grades of maple syrup: grade A light, medium, dark amber, and grade B, the darkest of all. There is no difference in quality between these grades, as they are used solely to distinguish the color and flavor of the syrup. As a general rule, the lighter the color, the earlier in maple season the syrup was made, and the milder the flavor.

Maple syrup is 90 percent sucrose, so it is rather like eating maple-flavored white sugar. Most of the vitamins and minerals are destroyed in the heating process.

Using Maple Syrup

Maple syrup can be used in a variety of recipes, including baked items like muffins and cakes. When using it in place of white sugar, you can substitute three quarters of a cup of maple syrup for one cup of sugar. Maple syrup should be stored in your refrigerator.

Safety Concerns

If you decide to use maple syrup, be sure to look for brands that are organic and guaranteed to be made without the use of formaldehyde, a toxic chemical commonly used in the production of most commercial brands of maple syrup.[26] Organic products tend to cost much more than the other brands, but this is also another indication that that it is actually organic.

Molasses

Molasses is considered a waste product of the sugar refining process. During the refining of sugarcane and sugar beets, the juice squeezed from these plants is boiled into a syrup mixture. Sugar crystals are then extracted from it. The brownish-black liquid that remains is molasses. But interestingly enough, the leftover "waste" consists mostly of the various nutrients that are naturally present in the cane juice. If the molasses is from sugarcane grown in high-quality soil, it will have some nutritional value.

Molasses is approximately 20–25 percent water, 50 percent sugar, and 10 percent mineral ash. The remaining components consist of protein and organic acids. Molasses is graded by color and sugar content. The lighter color types result from a shorter refining time and contain more sugar. The darker colors (i.e., blackstrap molasses) result from a longer refining process and, in turn, have less sugar and more nutrients and solids.

Paul Bergner, in his book *The Healing Power of Minerals*, recommends high-quality blackstrap molasses as a natural mineral supplement. It is especially high in iron, manganese, calcium, zinc, copper, and chromium, and also contains small amounts of potassium and magnesium.[27]

Using Molasses

Because of its very strong flavor, molasses is often used in baking, and is particularly useful in meat and vegetable dishes as a sweetener and coloring agent. You would typically use twice as much molasses as you would use honey in your baking recipes. It should be kept in a cool, dry place, or refrigerated.

Sucanat

Sucanat is advertised as a sweetener obtained by dehydrating the juice from organic sugarcane, thereby making it less processed and healthier. In actuality, though, it is sugar—sugar that is worse tasting because it contains molasses. It is also one of the most expensive alternative natural sweeteners and is 600 percent more costly than table sugar. Many companies who use Sucanat in their products do so because they simply want to avoid putting the word *sugar* on their ingredient labels, to trick the consumer into thinking that it is a healthier product.

Using Sucanat

Sucanat is brown in color, granular, and slightly less sweet than sugar. It has no additives or preservatives, dissolves readily in water, and can be used as a one-to-one replacement for other common sweeteners, including white sugar and brown sugar, although it seems to burn more easily with baking. Sucanat is typically available packaged, or in the bulk bins found in most health-food stores.[28]

Safety Concerns

The chemical make-up of Sucanat brand and table sugar are identical; therefore, Sucanat will have the same damaging effects as table sugar on your body. Sucanat brand may have slightly higher trace minerals because it contains some residual molasses, but not enough to be significant and justify the higher price.[29]

Please remember Sucanat is a brand name and is not a legal ingredient descriptor. The FDA Code of Federal Regulations requires that all ingredients must be listed by their common name to avoid confusion and any product extracted from sugarcane, like Sucanat, must be listed as "sugar" or "cane syrup," although this rule is frequently ignored by the food manufacturers.[30]

In summary, Sucanat is basically an expensive sugar . . . with very few additional nutritional benefits.

Turbinado Sugar

Turbinado sugar is highly refined and lacking a majority of the nutrients contained in honey or molasses. To give turbinado sugar a more natural look, a small amount of molasses is often mixed with the refined sugar to color it brown.[31] It's health risks are very similar to table sugar.

Further from the Tree

The term *natural* is a popular one these days. A progressively increasing number of people are searching for foods and other products that are wholesome and free of chemicals and preservatives. As I noted in chapter 5, many food companies have jumped on the "natural and organic" bandwagon and are attempting to benefit from this trend. As a result, a number of sweeteners have come into use recently that are claimed to be natural because of the substances from which they are derived. However, the fact that they are "derived" from anything suggests that they are processed and less than optimal.

The last few natural sweeteners I discussed included a number of products that also fall into the category of "derived." However, the processing required to create them is moderate and, for the most part, results in products that are still close to their original form.

The following list consists of a number of products that, for one reason or another, have fallen out of the realm of what I would consider natural. Nonetheless, most of them are still far better choices for you than artificial sweeteners, and safe for moderate consumption:

- Agave syrup
- Fructo-oligosaccharides (FOS)
- Fructose
- Fruit juice concentrate
- Sugar alcohols (Polyols)
- Tagatose

Agave Syrup, Agave Nectar

The agave plant is found in Mexico and contains a sweet, sticky juice. The ancient people of Mexico considered the plant to be sacred. When the Spaniards arrived, they fermented the agave juice to make tequila. Agave syrup is about 90 percent fructose. Some of the Internet sites selling agave syrup make the following claims about it:[32,33]

- Low glycemic index
- Delicious and safe alternative to table sugar
- Fifty percent sweeter than table sugar, yet has fewer calories per teaspoon
- Ideal for diabetics, hypoglycemics or those who cannot handle sucrose, and those watching their carb intake
- Supports normal intestinal function

Actually, none of this is true. To explain the truth about agave syrup requires a recounting of its history as a sweetener. In the early 1980s, blue agave was grown only for tequila and mescal distilling. Growers felt that they weren't making enough money selling agave at fifty dollars per U.S. ton, so they pooled their money to build a processing plant to convert it into hydrolyzed high-fructose inulin syrup (similar to HFCS). Then they introduced the new agave syrup in 1997 at the Anaheim Natural Foods Exposition, stating that it was an "all natural sweetener used since the Aztecs." They did not reveal that it was chemically converted fructose.

By this time, blue agave was overharvested and selling at an all-time high of $2,600 per ton. So naturally, the producers of the new agave syrup were asked how they were able to make it so inexpensively when 40 percent of the distilleries in Mexico had shut down because of the blue agave shortage. They responded that they were using other species of agave (there are 136 in all). When these species were investigated, however, they were directly linked to toxicity in humans; they cause breakdown of red blood cell membranes, and as little as two grams can cause spontaneous abortion in a pregnant woman.

The agave distributors have also been caught relabeling tankers of HFCS as agave syrup. When one of these distributors was caught doing this, one of the company officers stole all the assets and fled the country. After that incident, the FDA conducted an investigation of agave suppliers and decided how agave should be labeled as an ingredient. According to Title 21 of the Code of Federal Regulations all ingredients shall be listed by common name so that they do not mislead consumers. If the "principal constituent of agave is inulin . . . hydrolysis of inulin results in a syrup composed primarily of fructose. . . . The appropriate name for agave is 'hydrolyzed inulin syrup.'"

Although it is not legal per FDA mandate, agave syrup or products listing it on their label are readily available in health-food stores and on the Internet. The FDA doesn't have the staff or the manpower to go after the hundreds of thousands of small manufacturers in the health-food industry.

Is it dangerous? No one knows. It's impossible to tell if the product is derived from toxic agave plants, or is HFCS. But even if it's "only" hydrolyzed inulin syrup, that kind of processed fructose has all the adverse effects of sugar, plus it is more readily turned into triglycerides and fat than sucrose.

Avoid agave syrup.

SENOMYX

Senomyx, a biotech firm dedicated to taste receptor research, has created a taste potentiator chemicals that are able to activate or block taste receptors in the tongue and trick your brain into sensing a food is twice as salty or sweet than is really is. For instance, after adding only a few parts per million to a soda, the sugar content can be reduced by 40 percent but still taste the same. Several big food corporations, such as Kraft Foods, Nestlé, Coca-Cola, and Campbell Soup, are looking at adding these chemicals (the best one is known as Substance 951) to their foods.[34]

Because these taste potentiators will be used in tiny amounts (1 ppm), the FDA quickly gave it GRAS status after only a three-month rat study. It will be listed on labels as "artificial flavors."[35]

WARNING: Do you want to ingest an inadequately tested chemical designed to modulate your brain chemistry? What's next, are they going to put Prozac in your food to make you happier while you're eating their food?

Fructo-Oligosaccharides (FOS)

Fructo-oligosaccharides (abbreviated FOS) are a type of soluble fiber. FOS is not very sweet, so it is usually mixed with other, more intense sweeteners. Since FOS is also indigestible, it can cause gas, bloating, and other forms of digestive distress in some when eaten excessively.

Because of the widespread practice of mislabeling ingredients in the health-food industry, when you see FOS as an ingredient, there is a possibility that it is really fructose mislabeled in order to deceive you into believing the product is sugar-free.[36]

Fructose

Fructose is a naturally occurring sugar found in many foods, primarily fruit. However, when it is used as a sweetener in its powdered form, or as HFCS, it is highly processed. The fructose found as a sweetener in the ingredient lists of many products is typically refined from corn syrup or beet sugar. Because it breaks down at a slower rate in your body than sucrose does, fructose does not cause as much of a spike in your blood sugar, insulin, or leptin levels. It may sound like a better sweetener option than sugar, but it may in fact be one of the worst "natural" sweeteners of all. It is strongly recommended that you avoid this sweetener, as refined fructose has been shown to contribute to a number of the same problems as high-fructose corn syrup, which were discussed in chapter 1:[37-42]

- Excessive weight gain and obesity
- High triglyceride levels (blood fats)
- High blood pressure
- Insulin resistance
- Hyperglycemia
- Inflammation

Fruit Juice Concentrates

Concentrated fruit juice sweeteners are commonly used as the primary sweetener in many natural or organic products; therefore, you may believe that the product is healthy because it doesn't contain sugar. What you don't realize is that concentrated fruit juice sweeteners are a form of sugar and will cause identical problems that table sugar causes in your body. There are numerous peer-reviewed studies that document the harmful effects of fruit juice concentrates on the metabolism of infants and children, and pediatricians are encouraged to warn mothers to avoid providing excessive amounts of these chemically stripped juices to children.

Additionally, fruit juice concentrates have lost the majority of nutrients and fiber that are normally present in the fruit prior to processing. Some of these nutrients naturally oppose the effects that sugar has on your body, while the fiber in the fruit slows the absorption of the sugar from your digestive tract. Concentrates are also pasteurized, which destroys the valuable enzymes and beneficial phytonutrients found in whole raw fruits.

There is nowhere on the planet that you can find either fruit juice concentrate or fructose growing on a tree or bush. These highly processed products are a creation of modern technology; you were never designed to consume either of them. Fruit, on the other hand, has been around since ancient times. Although the domesticated forms we typically consume these days are higher in sugar than they used to be, fruit is still a far better alternative than refined fructose or fruit juice concentrate will ever be.

COMPARISON OF WHOLE FRUIT TO FRUIT CONCENTRATE:

Whole orange segments ½ cup	59 calories	14.4g carbs
Orange juice concentrate ½ cup	226 calories	54.2g carbs

If you really need to have something sweet, then a small piece of fruit would be a better option. If you are having consistent sweet cravings, there is a strong possibility you are not eating appropriately for your specific metabolic biochemistry, and it would be very helpful to learn more about Metabolic Typing on Mercola.com.

Sugar Alcohols (Polyols)

As their name suggests, sugar alcohols are, in fact, made from sugar. Scientists call them sugar alcohols because part of their structure chemically resembles sugar and part is similar to alcohol, but they don't completely fit into either category. Because of U.S. labeling laws, products containing sugar alcohols can, unfortunately, be labeled "Sugar-Free" when in fact they are on average only 50 percent fewer calories than sugar.

COMMON SUGAR ALCOHOLS (POLYOLS) AND THEIR CALORIC LOADS

SWEETENER	CALORIES PER GRAM
Sugar	4.0
Hydrogenated starch hydrolysates	3.0
Sorbitol	2.6
Xylitol	2.4
Maltitol	2.1

Isomalt	2.0
Lactitol	2.0
Mannitol	1.6
Tagatose	1.5
Erythritol	0.2

Sugar alcohols are used in a wide variety of low-calorie, reduced-calorie, low-fat, and sugar-free food applications, as they provide sweetness without contributing as many calories as sugar. These foods include baked goods, candy, gum, and frozen dairy desserts, among others.

If you are going to consume sugar alcohols, xylitol appears to be the best choice, as it has been associated with a variety of health benefits, such as preventing tooth decay and ear infections. Xylitol is used in toothpastes, mouthwashes, breath mints, and sprays, and pharmaceuticals such as cough syrups, cough drops, and throat lozenges.[43]

Safety Concerns

Sugar alcohols are found in very low levels in some raw fruits and vegetables, and do not cause problems in this natural state. However, the highly processed sugar alcohols used in the diet industry are very different from the ones found in nature.

Although sugar alcohols do not raise your blood sugar levels as much as table sugar, they do raise them. Sugar alcohols can also be converted to fat, and may contribute to an increase in blood triglyceride levels and weight gain.[44] The exception to this rule is erythritol, which does not appear to raise blood sugars but unfortunately also has inferior sweetening power.

A WARNING ABOUT "NET* CARBS"

There are numerous "low-carb" products on the market containing sugar alcohols as their sweeteners. You will often find the claim on snack bar labels, "Only 1 gram of net* carbs!" The back label, however, states that each bar actually has 19 or 20 grams of carbohydrates, but that these carbs don't count because they don't raise blood sugar levels.

According to Richard Bernstein, MD, author of the best-selling book *Dr. Bernstein's Diabetes Solution*, this is simply not the case: "Although it is true that sugar alcohols do not raise blood sugars as quickly or as much as sugar, they will still raise blood sugars and should be avoided by diabetics and anyone who is overweight."

For more advice on diabetes and health, see appendix D "What's a Diabetic to Do?"

Most sugar alcohols are *not* considered GRAS under food and beverage law, but they are allowed under American cosmetic, flavor, and pharmaceutical regulations. Be aware of polyol manufacturers who put the following phrases in their marketing literature and Web sites to convince you that the polyol is FDA approved: "This product has petitioned for self-affirmed GRAS status and has been accepted for filing by the U.S. FDA." Filing a petition and actually obtaining GRAS status are two entirely different standings.

Polyols can cause adverse digestive side effects including bloating, gastrointestinal distress, diarrhea, and anal leakage at moderate consumption levels of fifteen grams (1.5 teaspoons) per day.[45]

These detrimental side effects can also result in dehydration, equilibrium loss, vitamin and mineral depletion, malnutrition, and a higher vulnerability to disease. This can happen at lower dosage levels (as little as one gram, or .1 teaspoon, per day) in infants, children, diabetics, hyperinsulinemics or hypoglycemics, pregnant women, seniors, and many other health-compromised populations. Additionally, some polyols have been directly linked with malignant tumor activity.[46]

Maltitol, which is the most common sugar alcohol used in low-carb snack bars and chocolate, was denied GRAS petition status in 1994 by the FDA as a result of a significant number of laboratory animals contracting cancerous intestinal tumors in USDA-run tests, at relatively low ingestion levels.[47]

In 2000, the Center for Science in the Public Interest (CSPI) submitted a Citizen's Petition to the FDA, requesting mandatory product-warning labels for the use of any polyol. This petition's intent was to protect consumers from ingesting more than one gram of these ingredients, due to the high propensity of so many populations of consumers to have adverse digestive side effects.

Despite the potential for problems, I would still recommend xylitol over artificial sweeteners.

Tagatose (D-Tagatose)

Tagatose is fairly new to the sweetener market. The manufacturers of tagatose say that it is a naturally occurring substance found in heated dairy products, but processed tagatose is a very different molecule from the more natural version (not that heated dairy products are exactly natural). It is promoted as having the same chemical formula as fructose, but in fact the molecular structure for tagatose listed on its patent is that of a polyol. Once again, a false ingredient description is being used by the food industry to confuse the consumer.

Tagatose is not yet available in the United States as a ready-to-use sweetener, but it has been granted GRAS status by the FDA for use in beverages, cosmetics, processed foods, toothpastes, and medication. You may be able to find it on the label of some "sugar-free" items, probably listed as Naturalose™, the name used by its largest manufacturer, Spherix.

Health Benefit Claims

Tagatose is being marketed as a low-carbohydrate sweetener with numerous health benefits. Claims have been made about tagatose's ability to help reduce blood sugar spikes in diabetics, improve weight loss, and even fight cavities and bad breath. Some claims go even further, saying it can help prevent colon cancer or raise levels of HDL (good cholesterol) in your blood.[48] Although there is some reliability to the claims made about cavities, studies have yet to show consistent results regarding the others.[49]

Safety Concerns

Tagatose is no different from the other polyols with regard to safety concerns and has the same gastrointestinal side effects.

Don't Be Fooled by "Shugr™"

Recently, a "new" sweetener called Shugr has come on the market, billing itself as the "world's first natural, zero-calorie sweetener." But despite its "natural" claims, it is nothing but a blend of several of the sweeteners already discussed, including some highly processed ones and even artificial ones. It is composed of 99.5 percent tagatose, erythritol (another sugar alcohol), maltodextrin, and 0.5 percent sucralose.

Just Like Sugar® Lives Up To Its Name

Just Like Sugar is a popular new sugar substitute found in health food stores like Whole Foods. It contains inulin and chicory maltodextrin in the ingredients and claims not to raise blood sugars. (You should know by now that inulin and maltodextrin are both forms of sugar, so this claim is unlikely.) Dr. Bernstein, a type 1 diabetic, and Dr. Pearsall both tested their blood sugars with it, and it raised their blood sugars quite a bit—indeed just like sugar. In our opinion this product is being deceptively marketed and should be avoided as it is not much different than sugar and is more expensive.

SWEETENER COST COMPARISON*

Sweetener	Cost	Sweetener	Cost
Lo Han Kuo*	$2.80/oz.	Date Sugar	$0.37/oz.
Stevia*	$2.60/oz.	Barley Malt	$0.28/oz.
Equal	$1.14/oz.	Brown Rice Syrup (organic)	$0.23/oz.
Splenda	$0.91/oz.	Sucanat	$0.19/oz.
Agave Syrup	$0.81/oz.	Molasses	$0.18/oz.
Raw Honey	$0.75/oz.	Fruit Juice Concentrate	$0.17/oz.
Maple Syrup (organic)	$0.75/oz.	Turbinado	$0.16/oz.
Xylitol	$0.50/oz.	Fructose	$0.12/oz.
Sweet'N Low	$0.50/oz.	Sucrose (Table Sugar)	$0.03/oz.

*Bear in mind that Lo Han Kuo and stevia are comparatively expensive but are so much sweeter than the others that you would use much less.

"Organic"

Many of the products I have listed in this chapter can be bought with an "organic" label on them. Are they really organic? It's difficult to know for sure. Sometimes, the word *organic* on the label only means that the farmer paid four thousand dollars to buy an organic certification from the organic certifiers, because there isn't enough quality control to check these crops.[50] As much as reasonably possible, do as much research you can into how the foods you eat are produced.

The Bottom Line

Stevia appears to be the best choice as it is minimally processed, and like artificial sweeteners, it is hundreds of times sweeter than sugar so it has virtually no calories for the potency of it sweetening power. Although clearly sweet, not everyone enjoys its taste. Additionally it can not be sold as a sweetener in the United States, only as a dietary supplement.

Essentially, the biggest difference between most of the other sweeteners and table sugar is that they cost much more. The nutritional differences are minor. Still, I recommend that you try to use the ones that are the least processed and contain some minerals, like raw honey or molasses. If you choose to use table sugar, use cane instead of beet sugar because it is less processed.

Keep it simple. Reserve sweeteners for occasional use in small doses, and as long as you don't have serious challenges with controlling insulin levels, you should be fine.

CHAPTER NINE:
SWEET LIFE

THE PATH TO HEALTH

T he remainder of this book will provide you with the tools to avoid the dangers identified in the earlier chapters. Ideally, it should help you move toward a life where sweeteners and FDA safety regulations regarding food additives are simply no longer your concern.

Total Health Program

The previous chapters are an important introduction into my health program. Making changes to your diet and lifestyle may be one of the most difficult challenges you have ever faced. My earlier book, *Total Health Program*, was created as a practical tool to help you in this challenge.

In 1997, I started a free Internet health newsletter. The purpose of the newsletter was to use the Internet to educate the public and to catalyze the transformation of the fatally flawed medical paradigm. The Web site educates healthcare professionals and consumers to use lifestyle changes and natural remedies to restore health, instead of relying on drugs and surgery. Because there is a growing movement toward natural medicine, my newsletter eventually evolved into the number one natural health education Web site in the world: Mercola.com.

Every year my dedicated staff and I review tens of thousands of health articles and post the best ones on the site so that readers can be informed about the latest breakthroughs in how to achieve health. I was able to apply the best of this research in a clinical setting and revise them into powerful, simple, and inexpensive strategies that can help you obtain the optimal health that you were designed to enjoy.

In 2006, we plan on changing the site into Web 2.0 technology that will allow users to actively participate, rate, and comment on important health topics and create a treasure of health knowledge. If you have interest in participating in this exciting process, I encourage you to visit Mercola.com.

The *Total Health Program* provides a summary of the entire health and wellness program I've been using with my patients for the last twenty years. It condenses some of the most important principles from the over fifty thousand pages of free information that have been posted on Mercola.com. It also provides you with 150 recipes that follow my detailed and highly individualized dietary guidelines.

I hopefully have presented compelling evidence that you simply cannot trust the FDA, as they have strong ties to the very industries they are regulating. So where can you turn for reliable information about your food, your medications, and their real effects on your well-being?

If you want to identify trustworthy information sources, it is important to learn how to determine if an information source is credible. Most people, for example, do not question their physician's recommendations. If a drug is prescribed, they simply take it without hesitation.

But the majority of physicians (myself included) are trained in conventional medical schools that are funded and heavily influenced by the drug companies, where they are brainwashed into believing that the correct strategy for patient complaints is, nearly always, to prescribe some kind of expensive and potentially toxic drug.

It is well established that most medical schools provide very little practical training in nutrition, lifestyle coaching, or emotional healing. This is beginning to change, and Dr. Andrew Weil has been a positive force in this area, but there is still a long way to go. So it's no surprise that, when you visit most conventional physicians, you receive a drug prescription that merely addresses your symptoms and not the underlying cause of your problem.

There is a simple question you can ask yourself that will help guide your understanding as to whether or not the treatment being suggested will help you or hurt you:

"Is this treatment or recommendation addressing the *underlying cause* of my problem?"

Conversely, lifestyle changes and natural therapies are far more likely to solve the underlying cause, and do so with far less potential for harm.

Resources for General Health Information

Fortunately, you are not alone on your journey. There are a number of resources that can guide and assist you in the process of minimizing the artificial chemicals in your life. I have done my best in this book to inform you about some of the deceptions that the artificial sweeteners and the food industry use, but I have barely scratched the surface. However, living in the twenty-first century, you now also have the Internet as a tool that you can use to help you carefully investigate and discern the truth.

Once you have learned how to get past the media spin and understand the truth about these profoundly important health topics, you will develop a level of confidence that will help you defend your position against doubting relatives and friends who question your stance against conventionally accepted truths.

The following resources are offered as a suggestion as to where you can start or accelerate your lifelong journey to seek the truth:

Mercola.com

The Web site I started in 1997, Mercola.com, can serve as one of your primary resources. There are tens of thousands of health professionals and consumers alike who regularly use the site as a library that they go to when they have a specific question about natural health care.

Most people who visit Mercola.com regularly take advantage of the proactive drug warnings on the site. In 1999, I warned that Vioxx would eventually be removed from the market. This was well over one year before it was ever even approved, and five years before my prediction was realized. Over sixty thousand people died as a direct result of taking Vioxx. You can protect yourself by using the site to investigate the potential hazards of any medication you are taking or considering.

Additional Help from Mercola.com

The Web site is committed to helping you find inexpensive, nontoxic solutions to your health problems. The search engine on Mercola.com provides access to free information that can provide you with the practical tools to solve your health challenges.

Lab Testing Services—Our Newest Resource for You

Our newest resources are customized lab services. These allow you to accurately determine your lab values with a test that is covered by most insurance companies and is evaluated by a computer program that will give you detailed and specific instructions on how to improve your health based on your particular biochemistry.

I developed this computer program based on the lab results of the over ten thousand patients I have seen in my clinic and helped to recover their health. The information that this computer program generates can be used independently, or in conjunction with your local health-care provider. We hope to introduce the service in 2007.

In addition to Mercola.com, the following Web sites are recommended resources that you can trust for additional health information.

The Weston A. Price Foundation
westonaprice.org

The Weston A. Price Foundation is a nonprofit organization founded in 1999. Their goals are to provide accurate information on nutrition and human health, including the vital importance of animal fats in the diet, and to provide the resources and information necessary to help people transition to a natural way of eating. They derive the majority of their basic information from the research of Dr. Weston Price. Dr. Price spent years studying the lives, and especially the diets, of isolated nonindustrialized people, whom he found to be much healthier than the average citizen of more industrialized nations.

The Price Foundation uses research, education, and activism as a means of restoring a healthy diet to the general population. In their own words, they stand "united in the belief that modern technology should be harnessed as a servant to the wise and nurturing traditions of our ancestors rather than used as a force destructive to the environment and human health; and that science and knowledge can validate those traditions."

The Price-Pottenger Nutrition Foundation
price-pottenger.org

The Price-Pottenger Nutrition Foundation (PPNF) is another nonprofit organization whose main goal is to educate the public about the findings of Dr. Weston A. Price. They focus on disseminating the information gathered and researched by one of Price's better-known colleagues, Dr. Francis Pottenger. The discoveries of these two men have helped to form the basis of what we believe to be a truly healthy diet.

PPNF provides "accurate information on whole foods and proper preparation techniques, soil improvement, natural farming, pure water, non-toxic dentistry and holistic therapies in order to conquer disease; prevent birth defects; avoid personality disturbances & delinquency; enhance the environment; and enable all people to achieve long life and excellent health, now and into the twenty-first century."

Center for Science in the Public Interest
cspinet.org

The Center for Science in the Public Interest (CSPI) was established in 1971 as a national advocate for proper nutrition, food safety, alcohol policy, and sound scientific research. They have effected many positive health changes in the food industry.

Some of CSPI's past accomplishments include the following:

- A new federal law was enacted that sets standards for health claims on food labels and provides full and clear nutrition information on nearly all packaged foods (including the labeling of trans-fat per serving).

- Millions of Americans changed their food choices at popular restaurants thanks to CSPI's widely publicized studies on the nutritional value of restaurant meals; thousands of restaurants have added healthier options to their menus.

- Major fast-food chains have begun introducing healthier foods.

- Scores of deceptive ads by companies such as McDonald's, Kraft, and Campbell's Soup have been stopped.

Please note that I personally don't agree with all their nutritional positions, especially their stand against the use of saturated fat such as coconut oil, but I respect them for the work they are doing in battling industry.

Organic Consumers Organization
organicconsumers.org

"The Organic Consumers Association (OCA) is an online and grassroots non-profit public interest organization campaigning for health, justice, and sustainability. The OCA deals with crucial issues of food safety, industrial agriculture, genetic engineering, children's health, corporate accountability, Fair Trade, environmental sustainability and other key topics."

Acres USA
acresusa.com

Acres USA is dedicated to educating consumers and farmers about sustainable agriculture and food development practices, while providing an insider's view on the misguided practices of chemical farming. They provide an excellent magazine, online articles, and more.

American Association for Health Freedom (AAHF)
healthfreedom.net

AAHF was founded in 1992 in direct response to the problems faced by health care practitioners and consumers in the United States. AAHF works as an advocate to restore the medical freedoms that have been threatened by the U.S. Food and Drug Administration, the allopathic medical community, insurance companies, and state medical boards around the United States.

The Center for Food Safety (CFS)
centerforfoodsafety.org

The (CFS) is working to legally challenge harmful food production technologies and promote sustainable alternatives.

Early to Rise
earlytorise.com

Early to Rise offers an excellent newsletter that often goes behind the scenes of conventional business practices to provide you guidance on how to improve your health and well-being.

Environmental Working Group (EWG)
ewg.org

EWG specializes in environmental investigations. They have a team of scientists, engineers, policy experts, lawyers, and computer programmers who examine data from a variety of sources to expose threats to your health and the environment, and to find solutions.

The Fluoride Action Network
fluoridealert.org

The Fluoride Action Network is an international coalition seeking to broaden public awareness about the toxicity of fluoride compounds and the health impacts of current fluoride exposures. Along with providing comprehensive and up-to-date information on fluoride issues to citizens, scientists, and policymakers alike, FAN remains vigilant in monitoring government agency actions that may impact the public's exposure to fluoride.

Health Sciences Institute
hsibaltimore.com

The mission of the Health Sciences Institute, including their excellent newsletter, is to keep you informed of smart preventive health choices that will help you take control of your own health.

Nutrition for Optimal Health Association (NOHA)
nutrition4health.org

Providing information on healthier food choices and preventive health care, and dedicated to advancing scientific knowledge in the field of nutrition, NOHA presents lectures (usually based in the Chicago, IL area) and a quarterly newsletter.

Sustainable Table
sustainabletable.org

Sustainable Table promotes and educates consumers about making healthy food choices that support a sustainable system.

Union of Concerned Scientists
ucsusa.org

The Union of Concerned Scientists is the leading science-based nonprofit working for a health environment and a safer world. UCS combines independent scientific research and action to develop innovative, practical solutions and to secure responsible changes in government policy, corporate practices and consumer choices.

Conclusion

Seventy million Americans—almost a quarter of the entire population—currently have some form of cardiovascular disease; roughly a million die of it every year. Cancer has undergone a similar rapid increase, and in early

2005 surpassed heart disease as the leading cause of death in the United States for those under age eighty-five. Another seventy million Americans have diabetes or prediabetes; that is one in every four people in the United States. This is quite a change from the days when a busy doctor could see only two cases in his or her entire life.

If you are a typical American, your diet is slowly killing you.

Artificial sweeteners are perhaps the most extreme example of what has gone wrong with our eating habits. They are beyond processed; they are actually newly created chemicals produced in labs and factories. They serve no purpose other than to satisfy our addiction to something we don't really need to be eating in the first place. They are an attempt to cure our self-created illnesses, but they do nothing but create more disease.

This book may serve as a starting point in your journey to health. My impetus for writing it is that by learning about the dangers of artificial sweeteners, the companies that entice you to buy them, and the government that fails to protect you from them, you will begin to question the unnatural, dangerous food choices that have been thrust upon you since childhood.

It is my hope that you will become a diligent student of how you can continually improve your choices in your journey to achieve a high level health and wellness.

APPENDIX A

76 WAYS THAT SUGAR CAN
DESTROY YOUR HEALTH*

From *Lick the Sugar Habit* (Avery Publishing Group, 1996), by Nancy Appleton, PhD, www.nancyappleton.com

In addition to throwing off the body's homeostasis, excess sugar may result in a number of other significant consequences. The following is a listing of some of sugar's metabolic consequences from a variety of medical journals and other scientific publications:

1. Sugar can suppress your immune system and impair your defenses against infectious disease.[1,2]

2. Sugar upsets the mineral relationships in your body, causes chromium and copper deficiencies, and interferes with absorption of calcium and magnesium.[3-6]

3. Sugar can cause a rapid rise of adrenaline, hyperactivity, anxiety, difficulty concentrating, and crankiness in children.[7,8]

4. Sugar can produce a significant rise in total cholesterol, triglycerides, and bad cholesterol, and a decrease in good cholesterol.[9-12]

5. Sugar causes a loss of tissue elasticity and function.[13]

6. Sugar feeds cancer cells and has been connected with the development of cancer of the breast, ovaries, prostate, rectum, pancreas, biliary tract, lung, gallbladder, and stomach.[14-20]

7. Sugar can increase fasting levels of glucose and can cause reactive hypoglycemia.[21,22]

8. Sugar can weaken eyesight.[23]

9. Sugar can cause many problems with the gastrointestinal tract, including an acidic digestive tract, indigestion, malabsorption in patients with functional bowel disease, increased risk of Crohn's disease, and ulcerative colitis.[24-28]

10. Sugar can cause premature aging.[29]

11. Sugar can lead to alcoholism.[30]

12. Sugar can cause your saliva to become acidic, and can cause tooth decay and periodontal disease.[31-33]

13. Sugar contributes to obesity.[34]

14. Sugar can cause autoimmune diseases such as arthritis, asthma, and multiple sclerosis.[35-37]

15. Sugar greatly assists the uncontrolled growth of Candida Albicans (yeast infections).[38]

16. Sugar can cause gallstones.[39]

17. Sugar can cause appendicitis.[40]

18. Sugar can cause hemorrhoids.[41]

19. Sugar can cause varicose veins.[42]

20. Sugar can elevate glucose and insulin responses in oral contraceptive users.[43]

21. Sugar can contribute to osteoporosis.[44]

22. Sugar can cause a decrease in your insulin sensitivity, thereby causing abnormally high insulin levels and eventually diabetes.[45-47]

23. Sugar can lower your vitamin E levels.[48]

24. Sugar can increase your systolic blood pressure.[49]

25. Sugar can cause drowsiness and decreased activity in children.[50]

26. High sugar intake increases advanced glycation end products (AGEs—sugar molecules attaching to and thereby damaging proteins in the body).[51]

27. Sugar can interfere with your absorption of protein.[52]

28. Sugar causes food allergies.[53]

29. Sugar can cause toxemia during pregnancy.[54]

30. Sugar can contribute to eczema in children.[55]

31. Sugar can cause atherosclerosis and cardiovascular disease.[56,57]

32. Sugar can impair the structure of your DNA.[58]

33. Sugar can change the structure of protein and cause a permanent alteration of the way the proteins act in your body.[59,60]

34. Sugar can make your skin age by changing the structure of collagen.[61]

35. Sugar can cause cataracts and nearsightedness.[62,63]

36. Sugar can cause emphysema.[64]

37. High sugar intake can impair the physiological homeostasis of many systems in your body.[65]

38. Sugar lowers the ability of enzymes to function.[66]

39. Sugar intake is higher in people with Parkinson's disease.[67]

40. Sugar can increase the size of your liver by making your liver cells divide, and it can increase the amount of liver fat.[68,69]

41. Sugar can increase kidney size and produce pathological changes in the kidney, such as the formation of kidney stones.[70,71]

42. Sugar can damage your pancreas.[72]

43. Sugar can increase your body's fluid retention.[73]

44. Sugar is enemy number one of your bowel movement.[74]

45. Sugar can compromise the lining of your capillaries.[75]

46. Sugar can make your tendons more brittle.[76]

47. Sugar can cause headaches, including migraines.[77]

48. Sugar can reduce the learning capacity, adversely affect school children's grades, and cause learning disorders.[78,79]

49. Sugar can cause an increase in delta, alpha, and theta brain waves, which can alter your mind's ability to think clearly.[80]

50. Sugar can cause depression.[81]

51. Sugar can increase your risk of gout.[82]

52. Sugar can increase your risk of Alzheimer's disease.[83]

53. Sugar can cause hormonal imbalances such as increasing estrogen in men, exacerbating PMS, and decreasing growth hormone.[84–87]

54. Sugar can lead to dizziness.[88]

55. Diets high in sugar will increase free radicals and oxidative stress.[89]

56. High-sucrose diets for subjects with peripheral vascular disease significantly increases platelet adhesion.[90]

57. High sugar consumption by pregnant adolescents can lead to substantial decrease in gestation duration, and is associated with a twofold increased risk for delivering a small-for-gestational-age (SGA) infant.[91,92]

58. Sugar is an addictive substance.[93]

59. Sugar can be intoxicating, similar to alcohol.[94]

60. Sugar given to premature babies can affect the amount of carbon dioxide they produce.[95]

61. Decrease in sugar intake can increase emotional stability.[96]

62. Your body changes sugar into two to five times more fat in the bloodstream than it does starch.[97]

63. The rapid absorption of sugar promotes excessive food intake in obese subjects.[98]

64. Sugar can worsen the symptoms of children with attention deficit hyperactivity disorder (ADHD).[99]

65. Sugar adversely affects urinary electrolyte composition.[100]

66. Sugar can slow down the ability of your adrenal glands to function.[101]

67. Sugar has the potential of inducing abnormal metabolic processes in a normal healthy individual, and promoting chronic degenerative diseases.[102]

68. IVs (intravenous feedings) of sugar water can cut off oxygen to your brain.[103]

69. Sugar increases your risk of polio.[104]

70. High sugar intake can cause epileptic seizures.[105]

71. Sugar causes high blood pressure in obese people.[106]

72. In intensive care units, limiting sugar saves lives.[107]

73. Sugar may induce cell death.[108]

74. In juvenile rehabilitation camps, when children were put on a low-sugar diet, there was a 44 percent drop in antisocial behavior.[109]

75. Sugar dehydrates newborns.[110]

76. Sugar can cause gum disease.[111]

Used with permission.

APPENDIX B

LIST OF COMPLAINTS FILED AGAINST ASPARTAME WITH THE FDA (AS OF APRIL 1995)

The following list was compiled by the FDA based on roughly ten thousand consumer complaints regarding aspartame. Reported adverse reactions included (in order of frequency of report):

Headaches and migraines
Dizziness or problems with balance
Change in mood quality or level
Vomiting and nausea
Abdominal pain and cramps
Change in vision
Diarrhea
Seizures and convulsions
Memory loss
Fatigue, weakness
Other neurological problems
Rash
Sleep problems
Hives
Change in heart rate
Itching
Change in sensation (numbness, tingling)
Grand mal seizures
Local swelling
Change in activity level
Difficulty breathing
Oral sensory changes
Change in menstrual pattern
Other skin problems
Localized pain and tenderness
Other urogenital problems
Change in body temperature
Difficulty swallowing
Other metabolic problems
Joint and bone pain
Speech impairment
Other gastrointestinal problems
Chest pain
Other musculoskeletal problems
Fainting

Sore throat
Other cardiovascular problems
Change in taste
Difficulty with urination
Other respiratory problems
Edema
Change in hearing
Abdominal swelling
Change in saliva output
Change in urine volume
Change in perspiration pattern
Eye irritation
Muscle tremors
Petit mal seizures
Change in appetite
Change in body weight
Change in thirst or water intake
Unconsciousness and coma
Wheezing
Constipation
Other extremity pain
Problems with bleeding
Unsteady gait
Coughing
Blood glucose disorders
Blood pressure changes
Changes in skin and nail coloration
Change in hair or nails
Excessive phlegm production
Sinus problems
Simple partial seizures
Hallucinations
Shortness of breath from exertion
Blood in stool or vomit

Dysmenorrhea (painful menstrual cramps)
Dental problems
Change in smell
Death
Other blood or lymphatic problems
Eczema
Swollen lymph nodes
Hematuria (blood in urine)
Shortness of breath from position
Difficulties with pregnancy
Developmental retardation in children
Change in breast size or tenderness
Anemia
Change in sexual function
Shock
Conjunctivitis
Dilated eyes
Fever
Other or unspecified symptoms

APPENDIX C

RECOMMENDED FURTHER READING

Aspartame

Aspartame Disease: An Ignored Epidemic, by H. J. Roberts
This is a definitive book on reactions to aspartame. Dr. Roberts is widely regarded as the expert on aspartame disease because of his clinical experience and extensive research spanning two decades.

Sweet Misery: A Poisoned World (DVD)
(available on Mercola.com, mercola.com/2004/jul/24/sweet_misery.htm, or type in "Sweet Misery" on Google)
Sweet Misery is a compelling documentary of Cori Brackett's interviews across the country with medical and legal experts and victims of aspartame. Her drive to make the film was due to her own development of multiple sclerosis, which she attributes to drinking high of amounts of Diet Coke sweetened with aspartame. The film also goes into depth about the seedy politics involved in the FDA approval process for aspartame. This film is a must-see for anyone who uses aspartame.

The FDA

Hazardous to Our Health? FDA Regulation of Health-Care Products, by Robert Higgs
In this book, four outstanding scholars examine how the FDA accumulated its enormous power, and what effects it has had on the

public. It also explores who actually benefits and loses from FDA actions, and whether alternatives exist to safeguard the health of Americans.

The History of a Crime Against the Food Law, by Harvey Wiley (available of SweetDeception.com)

Harvey Wiley was the very first commissioner of the FDA, then known as the Bureau of Chemistry, and he was the driving force behind the passage of two landmark pieces of consumer protection legislation, the Pure Food and Drug Act and the Meat Inspection Act. This 1929 book is a description, by the person who would know best, of the government's frequent failure to enforce the Pure Food and Drug Act, and corruption in the early FDA.

The Food Industry

Food Fight: The Inside Story of the Food Industry, America's Obesity Crisis, and What We Can Do About It, by Kelly Brownell, PhD, and Katherine Horgen, PhD

Dr. Brownell, a professor at Yale and an expert on obesity, nutrition, and eating disorders, and coauthor Dr. Horgen trace the subtle convergence of public indifference, corporate opportunism, and tradition that in a few short decades has transformed the American waistline and created a tidal wave of disease. Drs. Brownell and Horgen outline bold public policy initiatives for reversing the trend, and describe steps individuals can take to help safeguard their own and their families' health.

Food Politics: How the Food Industry Influences Nutrition and Health, by Marion Nestle

As the former nutrition policy advisor to the FDA and Department of Agriculture, Marion Nestle was an insider to how the food industry influences nutrition and health in the United States. She gives numerous examples of this such as how the meat, dairy, and grain industries were able to influence the Food Pyramid and how food corporations exploit kids and corrupt the schools to sell their junk food.

Trust Us, We're Experts! How Industry Manipulates Science and Gambles with Your Future, by Sheldon Rampton and John Stauber
This book unmasks the sneaky and widespread methods industry uses to influence opinion through bogus experts, doctored data, and manufactured facts.

Natural Health Advice

Dr. Mercola's Total Health Program, by Dr. Joseph Mercola with Dr. Kendra Degen Pearsall, et al.
(available on Mercola.com at mercola.com/forms/total_health_book.htm)
If you could improve any aspect of your health today, what would you choose? Would you want to be at your ideal weight? Truly look and feel younger and avoid premature aging? Eliminate or vastly reduce some disease or illness? Increase your daily energy and not feel down or tired all the time? Something else, or all of the above? Imagine feeling healthier, full of energy, free of illness, and more upbeat throughout the day, no matter what your current condition. *Dr. Mercola's Total Health Program* is THE tool that will really help you make it happen, once and for all. The *Total Health Program* provides you with my entire clinically proven dietary and health program, including many health secrets that you haven't seen before. This is the same program that has so dramatically helped many thousands of patients at my clinic, The Optimal Wellness Center.

The Pharmaceutical Industry

The Truth About the Drug Companies: How They Deceive Us and What to Do About It, by Marcia Angell
During her two decades at the *New England Journal of Medicine,* Dr. Marcia Angell had a front-row seat for the appalling behavior of the pharmaceutical industry. Now, in this hard-hitting book, Dr. Angell

exposes the shocking truth of what the $200 billion pharmaceutical industry has become—and argues for essential, long-overdue change.

The Big Fix: How the Pharmaceutical Industry Rips Off American Consumers, by Katherine Greider

This meticulously reported expose uncovers exactly how the drug industry boosts sales and bilks consumers in the most lucrative prescription drug market in the world.

Stevia

The Stevia Cookbook: Cooking with Nature's Calorie-Free Sweetener, by Donna Gates and Dr. Ray Sahelian

This book includes documented studies and testimonials about stevia's safety, as well as more than one hundred recipes for entrées, side dishes, and desserts.

APPENDIX D

WHAT'S A DIABETIC (OR AN OVERWEIGHT PERSON) TO DO?*

Diabetics reading this book may be particularly upset over our recommendations to avoid artificial sweeteners. Artificial sweeteners seem like a perfect solution to help diabetics indulge their sweet tooth and still control their blood sugar. Even the American Diabetes Association recommends artificial sweeteners to diabetics. Unfortunately, after reading this book, you know they are not a wise choice at all. The following steps are helpful for diabetics to keep their blood sugars normal (80–95 mg/dl).

Step One: Earlier, in our description of the major ideas behind the *Total Health Program*, we discussed the necessity of *reducing or eliminating the use of sugar and grains in your diet.* This is the single most important change most diabetics can make. In addition, fine-tuning your diet with Metabolic Typing will provide you with some insights into the foods you can use to replace the grains and sugars.

Step Two: Use exercise as a tool to keep blood sugars in check. Exercise works by increasing the sensitivity of insulin and leptin receptors, so the insulin and leptin that you are already making works much more effectively to lower blood sugars. This eventually allows your body to reduce additional insulin and leptin production.

---

*This advice is not intended to replace that of your physician. We recommend that you consult with a physician before implementing any of the advice in this section. Although this section only addresses diabetes, most people who are overweight will have some degree of insulin and leptin resistance and have a high risk of developing diabetes. Those who are overweight would do well to follow the following advice given for diabetics, as the same treatment advice applies.

The more body fat you have, the higher the insulin and leptin resistance. The most effective way to decrease body fat is by increasing muscle mass with weight training. Aerobic exercise is also important. Please note that diabetics with blood sugars over 170 mg/dl need to use extra caution and medical supervision for their exercise program, because elevated blood sugars may rise further with exercise.

Most people don't recognize the importance of exercise intensity. They don't understand that gentle walking, even for ninety minutes, isn't a sufficiently intense exercise. You need to go hard enough so that you would have a difficult time talking to someone, and then drop back half a notch. If you can easily carry on a conversation with someone next to you, then you are going too slowly to generate the aerobic benefits that exercise is capable of providing.

One of the key principles is to listen to your body. If your body will not allow you to exercise, either due to pain or worsening of your underlying condition, then you have no practical option but to honor your body's signals and not exercise. Even though your body desperately needs the exercise to improve, you will only get worse if you violate your current limitations. So you may have to start with as little as one or two minutes a day. Apply the *Total Health Program*, and as your body gradually improves, so will your exercise tolerance.

Step Three: Be sure to *get enough (but not too much) sleep*, as studies have shown that sleeping five hours or less or nine hours or more each night may increase your risk of developing diabetes.[1] In this country we have an epidemic of people who are sleep deprived. The average American is only getting seven hours of sleep, when s/he should be getting eight to nine. Additionally, many people also struggle with insomnia. If you are one of the 58 percent of Americans who struggle with getting a full night of sleep, we suggest reading *The Guide to a Good Night's Sleep*, available free at Mercola.com.

Read *Dr. Bernstein's Diabetes Solution*, by Richard Bernstein, MD

This book covers what a diabetic needs to know to manage their diabetes using a low-carbohydrate diet. It includes dietary recommendations similar to those given in the *Total Health Program*, but with a very strict regulation of carbohydrate intake.

The book also gives information on blood sugar testing, lab tests, supplies, how to prevent hypoglycemia, exercise routines, avoidance of complications, and even how to properly use insulin when necessary. The only caveat is that he advocates artificial sweeteners.

APPENDIX E

THE ORIGINS OF SWEETENERS

The only concentrated sugar that early man would have had access to was honey. But research of modern-day hunter-gatherers shows that the average honey consumption was minor—maybe four pounds, or 3 percent of total calories, over the course of an entire year.[1,2]

Cave paintings in Spain from 7000 B.C. show that beekeeping began quite early. Honey was prized and revered in ancient Egypt, Greece, and Rome—beekeeping was a major industry throughout the Roman Empire.[3] But the ability to produce concentrated sugar on a truly massive scale didn't exist until the invention of sugarcane processing.

Sugarcane is one of the oldest agricultural crops in the world, first cultivated in Papua New Guinea (an island north of Australia) perhaps nine thousand years ago. From there it spread to India around 500 B.C. and China around 250 B.C. But at that time, it was just a mildly sweet, woody plant—sugar was extracted in small quantities by chewing and sucking on the cane.

It was not until A.D. 500 that the Indians introduced commercial sugar extraction by pressing out the juice and boiling it into crystals. By A.D. 600, this practice had become widespread. During the Muslim expansion in the seventh century, Arabs invaded Persia and learned the coveted secret of sugar production. In the eleventh century, when the crusaders came pillaging through the Muslim's territory, they discovered sugar and carried it back to Europe, where it caused a sensation. The demand for sugar caused a dramatic increase in trade between western Europe and Eastern Europe.[4]

But sugar production was labor intensive, and therefore expensive to produce. The extensive costs to produce sugar made it a luxury item, frequently referred to as "white gold" (the price of a kilo in London in 1319 was the equivalent of *one hundred dollars* at today's prices!⁵). This effectively restricted the use of sugar to all but the very wealthy.

Sugar and Slavery

The sugar industry experienced a revolutionary shift after Christopher Columbus arrived in the New World. When Columbus sailed to the Caribbean islands in 1492, he planted sugarcane, which thrived in the favorable climate. So he took the natives' land and forced them into slavery to cultivate the sugarcane. But most of the natives died from the European diseases, overwork, or execution, so they were replaced by African slaves and European indentured servants.

> Queen Elizabeth I of England (1533–1603) was so fond of eating sugar that she had extensive dental decay, which caused all her teeth to rot and turn black. In all of her portraits, her mouth is closed.

In modern America, we tend to think of cotton plantations as the driving economic force behind slavery. But in fact, historical documents make it quite clear that without sugar, the slave trade would have been relatively minor. Sugar and the slave trade were a foundation of the European marketplace. African slavery was the main factor that radically changed the economics of the sugar industry and was able to reduce the cost of sugar from the one-hundred-dollars-per-kilo price in 1319 to the equivalent of six dollars per kilo by 1500. Finally, sugar was inexpensive enough for the average person to use. Between 1663 and 1775, English use of sugar increased *twentyfold*, and nearly all of it was produced in the Americas.

This radical reduction in the cost of sugar came at the expense of the slaves who were kidnapped from Africa. The typical slave had an average life span of ten years after arriving in the West Indies. The work was brutal, and slaves were forced to labor eighteen hours a day during the harvest season. A typical daily food ration was only one fish and nine plantains.

The late seventeen hundreds saw the rise of the emancipation movement. Along with the idealists who wished to spread liberty, the movement was in part funded by sugar companies who used hired help in India and wanted to turn the public against the slave-based competition. Slavery in the West Indies was abolished by Britain in 1833, although they did not enforce it until 1837. But the sugar plantation owners did everything in their power to force the emancipated slaves back into slavery: They charged high rents so the former slaves could not afford to live. They created laws that, if violated, would force the convicts into slavery. They burned down the villages of former slaves that were located too far from the plantations, in order to bring them back under their control.[6]

In the early eighteen hundreds, during the Napoleonic wars, there was a blockade that cut off continental Europe from cane sugar importation. Napoleon had heard about technology used to extract sugar from the sugar beet and declared that sugar would be produced from beets from that point forward. Sugarcane growers began to face stiff competition as sugar prices plunged worldwide. Since that time, the sugar cane and sugar beet companies have been fierce competitors.

Records from the 1700s describe the unappetizing art of sugar production. To begin, the sugar was treated with lime water and then a clearing medium was added—the most popular being two gallons of bull's blood or eighty egg whites (wood ash, milk, charcoal, lime, sulfurous acid, carbon dioxide, alum, and lead acetate have also been used at various times).

The cane growers who survived were those who managed to find cheap labor and bring in machinery to increase efficiency. Peasants from India, China, and Japan were brought in to meet the labor demands. Due to the high incidence of diseases such as yellow fever and malaria, the death rates were just as high for these peasant laborers as they were for the African slaves.

The plunging prices of sugar caused consumption to dramatically increase. Over the course of the nineteenth century, the English would up their sugar consumption once again, this time fivefold.[7]

But this fivefold increase is nothing compared to what we eat today—an increase of 469 times since the 1800s. The world as a whole is addicted to sugar.

The Increase in Worldwide Sugar Production Over Time[e]

(One ton = 2,204 pounds. An eighteen-wheeler truck weighs two tons.)

Year	Tons per Year
• 1800:	245,000
• 1830:	800,000
• 1900:	8 million
• 1975:	80 million
• 2004:	115 million

Very few foods in the history of the world have seen such explosive growth in production and consumption.

APPENDIX F

CODE OF FEDERAL REGULATIONS
TITLE 21, VOLUME 2

[Code of Federal Regulations]
[Title 21, Volume 2]
[Revised as of April 1, 2001]
From the U.S. Government Printing Office via GPO Access
[CITE: 21CFR102.5]

[Page 171-172]

TITLE 21—FOOD AND DRUGS

CHAPTER I—FOOD AND DRUG ADMINISTRATION, DEPARTMENT OF HEALTH AND HUMAN

SERVICES—CONTINUED

PART 102—COMMON OR USUAL NAME FOR NONSTANDARDIZED FOODS—Table of Contents

Subpart A—General Provisions

Sec. 102.5 General principles. http://www.cfsan.fda.gov/~lrd/CFR102-5.HTML

(a) The common or usual name of a food, which may be a coined term, shall accurately identify or describe, in as simple and direct terms as possible, the basic nature of the food or its characterizing properties or ingredients. The name shall be uniform among all identical or similar products and may not be confusingly similar to the name of any other food that is not reasonably encompassed within the same name. Each class or subclass of food shall be given its own common or usual name that states, in clear terms, what it is in a way that distinguishes it from different foods. (b) The common or usual name of a food shall include the percentage(s) of any characterizing ingredient(s) or component(s) when the proportion of such ingredient(s) or component(s) in the food has a material bearing on price or consumer acceptance or when the labeling or the appearance of the food may otherwise create an erroneous impression that such ingredient(s) or component(s) is present in an amount greater than is actually the case. The following requirements shall apply unless modified by a specific regulation in subpart B of this part.

(1) The percentage of a characterizing ingredient or component shall be declared on the basis of its quantity in the finished product (i.e., weight/weight in the case of solids, or volume/volume in the case of liquids).

(2) The percentage of a characterizing ingredient or component shall be declared by the words "containing (or contains) __ percent (or %) _____" or "__ percent (or %) _____" with the first blank filled in with the percentage expressed as a whole number not greater than the actual percentage of the ingredient or component named and the second blank filled in with the common or usual name of the ingredient or component. The word "containing" (or "contains"), when used, shall appear on a line immediately below the part of the common or usual name of the food required by paragraph (a) of this section. For each characterizing ingredient or component, the words "__ percent or %) _____" shall appear following or directly below the word "containing" (or contains), or directly below the part of the common or usual name of the food required by paragraph (a) of this section when the word "containing" (or contains) is not used, in easily legible boldface print or type in distinct contrast to other

printed or graphic matter, and in a height not less than the larger of the following alternatives:

(i) Not less than one-sixteenth inch in height on packages having a principal display panel with an area of 5 square inches or less and not less than one-eighth inch in height if the area of the principal display panel is greater than 5 square inches; or (ii) Not less than one-half the height of the largest type appearing in the part of the common or usual name of the food required by paragraph (a) of this section. (c) The common or usual name of a food shall include a statement of the presence or absence of any characterizing ingredient(s) or component(s) and/or the need for the user to add any characterizing ingredient(s) or component(s) when the presence or absence of such ingredient(s) or component(s) in the food has a material bearing on price or consumer acceptance or when the labeling or the appearance of the food may otherwise create an erroneous impression that such ingredient(s) or component(s) is present when it is not, and consumers may otherwise be misled about the presence or absence of the ingredient(s) or component(s) in the food. The following requirements shall apply unless modified by a specific regulation in subpart B of this part. (1) The presence or absence of a characterizing ingredient or component shall be declared by the words "containing (or contains) _____" or "containing (or contains) no _____" or "no _____" or "does not contain _____," with the blank being filled in with the common or usual name of the ingredient or component.

(2) The need for the user of a food to add any characterizing ingredient(s) or component(s) shall be declared by an appropriate informative statement.

(3) The statement(s) required under paragraph (c)(1) and/or (2) of this section shall appear following or directly below the part of the common or usual name of the food required by paragraphs (a) and (b) of this section,

in easily legible boldface print or type in distinct contrast to other printed or graphic matter, and in a height not less than the larger of the alternatives established under paragraphs (b)(2) (i) and (ii) of this section.

(d) A common or usual name of a food may be established by common usage or by establishment of a regulation in subpart B of this part, in part 104 of this chapter, in a standard of identity, or in other regulations in this chapter.

ACKNOWLEDGMENTS

Without a doubt this has been the most challenging book I have ever written, and it has taken more than two years to compile a strong case that would stand up to the scrutiny that will be directed at it.

I would like to thank the people that were directly involved in making this book happen.

My coauthor, Dr. Pearsall, played a crucial role with this book; in addition to her research, writing, and editing, she assembled and managed our team of researchers, technical experts, and editors, and secured the challenging critical pieces that are necessary to compile an exposition of this magnitude. She also worked tirelessly for an entire year of writing and endless revisions that were required.

Without her I would never have found Ry Herman, who did a masterful job on the editing of the book. I am very grateful to have had his assistance.

Researchers who helped compile much of the initial research: One of them was Dr. Daniel Chong, and the others wish to remain anonymous.

Dr. Richard Bernstein pointed out some critical issues such as the fact that 96 percent of the material in an artificial packet is pure sugar.

Several industry experts, who wish to remain anonymous because they are afraid of retribution, must be thanked also.

Thank you to Dr. Betty Martini, for volunteering countless hours of research and editing for the book and for her selfless devotion to helping victims of artificial sweetener poisoning with her Web sites www.dorway.com and www.wnho.net.

NOTES

FOREWORD

1. DAMS Inc., Mercury Free and Healthy, August 2005, http://www.amalgam.org/#anchor59579.
2. Richard Harkness, "Mercury in Flu Shot No Danger," *Citizen*, March 2005, http://www.thecitizen.com/archive/main/archive-050302/pt-05_mercury.html.
3. Manette Loudon, "Prescription Drug Alert: Millions at Risk from Serious and Possibly Deadly Side Effects," *Crusador* 25 (June/July 2005), http:// www.mercola.com/2005/aug/13/secrets_of_the_fda_revealed_by_top_insider_doctor.htm.
4. *San Francisco Chronicle*, January 2, 1970.
5. Testimony before the House Subcommittee on Intergovernmental Relations, 1970.
6. Minutes of the Proprietary Association Convention, White Sulphur Springs, Virginia, 1949.
7. Hearings of the Senate Subcommittee on Administrative Practice and Procedure, 1965.

CHAPTER ONE

1. R. Audette and T. Gilchrist, *NeanderThin: Eat Like a Caveman to Achieve a Lean, Strong, Healthy Body* (New York: St. Martin's Press, 1999).
2. Ibid.
3. W. Price, *Nutrition and Physical Degeneration*, 17th ed. (La Mesa: Price-Pottenger Nutrition Foundation, Inc., 2006).
4. B. Meehan, *Shell Bed to Shell Midden* (Canberra, Australia: Humanities Press, 1982).
5. K. Hawkes, K. Hill, and J. F. O'Connell, "Why Hunters Gather: Optimal Foraging and the Ache of Eastern Paraguay," *American Ethnologist* 9 (1982): 379-98.
6. P. Macinnis, *Bittersweet: The Story of Sugar* (Crows Nest: Allen & Unwin, 2002).
7. "Table 52—High fructose corn syrup: estimated number of per capita calories consumed daily, by calendar year." ers.usda.gov/briefing/sugar/data.htm
8. R. Marz, *Medical Nutrition from Marz*, 2nd ed. (Portland: Omni-Press, 1997).
9. D, Kirschenbaum, *The 9 Truths About Weight Loss: The No- Tricks, No-Nonsense Plan for Lifelong Weight Control* (New York: Owl Books, 2001), 56.
10. "Sugar Intake Hit All-time High in 1999," May 18, 2000, http://www.scpinet.org/new/sugar_limit.html.
11. Ibid.

12. M. Jacobson, "Liquid Candy: How Soft Drinks Are Harming Americans' Health," http://www.cspinet.org/new/pdf/liquid_candy_final_w_new_supplement.pdf.

13. M Nestle. *Food Politics: How the Food Industry Influences Nutrition and Health* (Berkeley: University of California Press, 2002)

14. Jacobson, "Liquid Candy."

15. M. Gibney, M. Sigmam-Grant, Dr. Keast. "Consumption of Sugars." *American Journal of Clinical Nutrition* 62, suppl. (1995): 178S–94S.

16. John Sicher, "Beverage Digest/Maxwell Ranks U.S. Soft Drink Industry for 2004," press release, *Beverage Digest*, March 4, 2005, http://www.beverage-digest.com/pdf/top-10_2005.pdf.

17. M. Eades and M. Eades, *Protein Power* (New York: Bantam, 1996).

18. R. Bernstein, *Dr. Bernstein's Diabetes Solution: The Complete Guide to Achieving Normal Blood Sugars* (Boston: Little Brown & Company, 2003).

19. N. Appleton, *Lick The Sugar Habit* (Garden City Park: Avery Publishing Group, 1996)

20. W. Ringsdorf, E. Charaskin, and E. Ramsey, "Sucrose Neutrophilic Phagocytosis and Resistance to Disease," *Dental Survey* 52 no. 12 (1976): 46–48.

21. W. Glinsmann, H. Irausquin, and Y. Park, "Evaluation of Health Aspects of Sugars Contained in Carbohydrate Sweeteners," FDA Report of Sugars Task Force, 1986, 39.

22. Appleton, *Lick the Sugar Habit.*

23. S. Elliott, N. Keim, J. Stern, K. Teff, and P. Havel, "Fructose, Weight Gain, and the Insulin Resistance Syndrome," *American Journal of Clinical Nutrition* 76, no. 5 (November 2002): 911–22.

24. G. Bray, S. Nielsen, and B. Popkin, "Consumption of High-Fructose Corn Syrup in Beverages May Play a Role in the Epidemic of Obesity," *American Journal of Clinical Nutrition* 79, no. 4 (2004): 537–43.

25. S. Kleiner, "The Devil's Candy," *Men's Health Magazine*, 2003, my.webmd.com.

26. "BMI–Body Mass Index: BMI Calculator," www.cdc.gov.

27. C. Cowie, K. F. Rust, D. D. Byrd-Holt et al., "Prevalence of Diabetes and Impaired Fasting Glucose in Adults in the U.S. Population," National Health and Nutrition Examination Survey 1999–2002, Diabetes Care 29 (June 2006): 1263-1268.

28. CDC, "National Diabetes Fact Sheet," www.cdc.gov/diabetes/pubs/pdf/ndfs_2005.pdf.

29. International Diabetes Federation, "Diabetes Deaths to Increase Dramatically over Next Ten Years," 2005, www.idf.org/home/index.cfm?unode=7952D720-102D-4842-8487-FB94FEC5B275.

30. Macinnis, *Bittersweet.*

ADDITIONAL CHAPTER ONE REFERENCES

American Diabetes Association. "Evidence-Based Nutrition Principles and Recommendations for the Treatment and Prevention of Diabetes and Related Complications." *Diabetes Care* 25 (2002): 202–12. care.diabetesjournals.org.

Centers for Disease Control. "Overweight and Obesity." June 2004. www.cdc.gov.

The Cleveland Clinic. "Weight Loss: Health Risks Associated with Obesity." August 2004. my.webmd.com.

Economic Research Service, USDA. "Caloric and Low-Calorie Sweeteners Per Capita Consumption." 2004. ers.usda.gov.

J. Hallfrisch, "Metabolic Effects of Dietary Fructose." *Federation of American Societies for Experimental Biology* 4 (June 1990): 2652–60.

G. Mirkin, "Advanced Glycation End Products." 2000. www.drmirkin.com.

D. Schwarzbein, *The Schwarzbein Principle II: The Transition* (Deerfield Beach: Health Communications, Inc., 2002)

B. Sears, *The Anti-Aging Zone* (New York: Regan Books, 1998)

CHAPTER TWO

1. CDC, "Toxicological Profile for Toluene," www.atsdr.cdc.gov.

2. W. Duke, "Saccharin: A Real Look at an Artificial Sweetener," web1.caryacademy.org.

3. C. Fahlberg and I. Remsen, "Ueber die Oxydation des Orthotoluolsulfamids," *Chemische Berichte* 12 (1879): 469–73.

4. W. Brody, "Biomedical Engineering Lecture Series: From Minds to Minefields: Negotiating the Demilitarized Zone Between Industry and Academia," [source?] 1999.

5. Ibid.

6. P. Macinnis, *Bittersweet: The Story of Sugar* (Crows Nest: Allen & Unwin, 2002).

7. Ibid.

8. M. W. Wagner, "Cyclamate Acceptance," *Science* 168 (1970): 1605.

9. I. F. Gaunt, M. Sharratt, P. Grasso, A. B. Lansdown, and S. D. Gangolli, "Short-Term Toxicity of Cyclohexylamine Hydrochloride in the Rat," *Food and Cosmetics Toxicology* 12, nos. 5–6 (October 1974): 609–24.

10. R. W. James, R. Heywood, and D. Crook, "Testicular Responses of Rats and Dogs to Cyclohexylamine over Dosage," *Food and Cosmetics Toxicology* 3, no. 19 (June 1981): 291–96.

11. A. Roberts and A. G. Renwick, "The Pharmacokinetics and Tissue Concentrations of Cyclohexylamine in Rats and Mice," *Toxicology and Applied Pharmacology* 2, no. 98 (April 1989): 230–42.

12. A. Roberts, A. G. Renwick, G. Ford, D. M. Creasy, and I. Gaunt, "The Metabolism and Testicular Toxicity of Cyclohexylamine in Rats and Mice During Chronic Dietary Administration," *Toxicology and Applied Pharmacology* 2, no. 98 (April 1989): 216–29.

13. http://www.fda.gov/bbs/topics/ANSWERS/ANS00155.html.

14. S. Fukushima, M. Arai, J. Nakanowatari, T. Hibino, M. Okuda, and N. Ito, "Differences in Susceptibility to Sodium Saccharin Among Various Strains of Rats and Other Animal Species," *Gann* 74 (February 1983): 8–20.

15. J. M. Taylor, M. A. Weinberger, and L. Friedman, "Chronic Toxicity and Carcinogenicity to the Urinary Bladder of Sodium Saccharin in the In Utero-Exposed Rat," *Toxicology and Applied Pharmacology* 1, no. 54 (June 1980): 57–75.

16. R. A. Squire, "Histopathological Evaluation of Rat Urinary Bladders from the IRDC Two-Generation Bioassay of Sodium Saccharin," *Food and Chemical Toxicology* 23, nos. 4–5 (April–May 1985): 491–97.

17. Duke, "Saccharin: A Real Look at an Artificial Sweetener."

18. R. Powelson, "Warnings No Longer Required for Products Containing Saccharin," *Nando Media*, January 2001, April 2001, www.nandotimes.com.

19. "The Delaney Clause" at: ipm.ncsu.edu/safety/factsheets/delaney.pdf#search=22 delaney%20clause%2220.

20. Burkhard Bilger, "The Search for Sweet," *The New Yorker*, May 22, 2006.

21. Federal Register, December 31, 2003, vol. 68, no. 250, Rules and Regulations, 75411-75413, http://www.cfsan.fda.gov/~lrd/fr031231.html; from the Federal Register Online via GPO Access, wais.access.gpo.gov, DOCID:fr31de03-15.

22. Department of Health and Human Services, Food and Drug Administration.

23. CFR Part 172, Docket no. 2002F-0220, "Food Additives Permitted for Direct Addition to Food for Human Consumption; Acesulfame Potassium," AGENCY: Food and Drug Administration, HHS, ACTION: Final rule.

24. http://www.cfsan.fda.gov/~lrd/fr031231.html; Aspartame Controversy in 1988:

   a) UPI, http://www.dorway.com/upipaper.txt; Gregory Gordon, UPI Investigative Report, "NutraSweet: Questions Swirl. Part 1: Did Searle Ignore Early Warning Signs?" 1987.

   b) Congressional Hearings: U.S. Senate 1987. U.S. Senate Committee on Labor and Human Resources, November 3, 1987, regarding "NutraSweet Health and Safety Concerns," Document # Y 4.L 11/4:S.HR6.100.

25. M. Jacobson, "Artificial Sweetener 'Sunett' Should Not Be Used in Diet Soda, New Tests Needed, Cancer Experts Tell FDA," 1996, www.cspinet.org/new/ask.html.com, accessed June 26, 2006. Sample quotes from cancer experts' letters on acesulfame testing, http://www.cspinet.org/foodsafety/additives_acesulfame.html.

26. M. Jacobson, L. Lefferts, and A. Garland, *Safe Food* (Berkley, CA: Berkley Publishing Group, 1991).

27. "Sugar Substitutes—Are They Safe?" ag.arizona.edu.

28. D. Woods, "U.S. Scientists Challenge Approval of Sweetener." *BMJ*, 313, 386 (August 17, 1996).

29. "Cost Is the Key to Neotame's Success," Food Navigator-USA.com, 2005, www.food navigator-usa.com/news-by-product/news.asp?id=58489&idCat=88&k=cost-is-the.

30. "Facts on Toxicity, Safety and Usage for Neotame," www.neotame.com.

31. J. Samuels, "For Better or Worse," www.truthinlabeling.org/forB.html.

ADDITIONAL CHAPTER TWO REFERENCES

Bachmanov, A. A., M. G. Tordoff, and G. K. Beauchamp. "Sweetener Preference of C57BL/6ByJ and 129P3/J Mice." *Chemical Senses* 7, no. 26 (September 2001): 905–13.

Brewer, Susan M., and Miriam Edlefsen. "National Food Safety Database: Saccharin." August 2000. www.foodsafety.ufl.edu.

"Coca Cola C2, Ingredients and Nutrition List," www.bevnet.com.

Corporatewatch.org Web site, www.corporatewatch.org.uk.

FoodProcessing.com Web site, www.foodprocessing.com.

John Fry, Director, Connect Consulting, Stratecon International Consultants.

Giles, Bridget, ed. *Inventions & Inventors*. New York: Grolier Educational, 2000: 57–58.

Greenberg, Lowell J. *Saccharin: Symbol of Our Age*. March 2001, April 2001.

James, Peter, and Nick Thorpe, *Ancient Inventions* New York: Ballantine Books, 1995: 304–5.

Kestler, Daryl, ed. "Artificial Sweeteners." *Nutrition and Fitness*. New York: Macmillan Reference, 1995.

Lagowski, Joseph. "Sweeteners." *Encyclopedia of Chemistry*. New York: Macmillan Reference, 1997.

Liang, Y., G. Steinbach, V. Maier, and E. F. Pfeiffer. "The Effect of Artificial Sweetener on Insulin Secretion"; "The Effect of Acesulfame-K on Insulin Secretion in the Rat (Studies In Vivo)." [both articles in same publ] *Hormone and Metabolic Research* 6, no. 19 (June 1987): 233–38.

McGrath, Kimberley A., ed. "Artificial Sweetener." *World of Invention*, 2nd ed. Detroit: Gale Research, 1999.

Mukherjee, A., and J. Chakrabarti. "In Vivo Cytogenetic Studies on Mice Exposed to Acesulfame-K—a Non-Nutritive Sweetener." *Food Chemistry Toxicology* [should this be Food and Chemical Toxicology? Found that written out in another note] 12, no. 35 (December 1997): 1177–79.

"NTP Chemical Repository: Saccharin," ntp-server.niehs.nih.gov.

Powers, M. A. "Sweetener Blending: How Sweet It Is!" *Journal American Dietetic Association* 94 (May 1994): 498.

Ronzio, Robert A., PhD. "Artificial Sweeteners." *The Encyclopedia of Nutrition and Good Health*. New York: Facts on File, Inc, 1997.

Ronzio, Robert A., PhD. "Saccharin." *The Encyclopedia of Nutrition and Good Health*. New York: Facts on File, Inc, 1997.

Roosevelt, Theodore. "Peace Commission at Portsmouth." 2001.

"Saccharin: Symbol of Our Age," earthrenewal.org

Stolberg, Sheryl Gay. "Bid to Absolve Saccharin Is Rebuffed by U.S. Panel," *New York Times*. 1997.

Sweet One Web site, sweetone.com.

Women.com Networks, Inc. "Nutrition and Diet: Saccharin." 2001.

CHAPTER THREE

1. Cori Brackett and J. T. Waldron, *Sweet Misery: A Poisoned World* (Sound and Fury Productions, 2004).

2. H. J. Roberts, *Aspartame Disease: An Ignored Epidemic* (West Palm Beach: Sunshine Sentinel Press, 2001).

3. Brackett and Waldron, *Sweet Misery: A Poisoned World*.

4. Study E-33, 34, Cross Reference E-87, Master File 134 for Aspartame, FDA Hearing Clerk's Office.

5. Gordon, Gregory, UPI investigative report, "NutraSweet: Questions Swirl," October 12, 1987. Reprinted in U.S. Senate, 1987, 483-510, http://www.dorway.com/upipaper.txt.

6. Citation for Helling memo: Herbert Helling, 1970. Memorandum from Herbert

Helling, G.D. Searle Official to several G.D. Searle Officials, regarding Food and Drug Sweetener Strategy, December 28, 1970, Reprinted in U.S. Senate Joint Hearings before the Subcommittee on Health of the Committee on Labor and Public Welfare and the Subcommittee on Administrative Practice and Procedure of the Committee on the Judiciary, "Preclinical and Clinical Testing by the Pharmaceutical Industry, 1976, Part 2," no. Y4.L11/2:P49/2/976/pt2, CIS# S541-82, 16–19.

7. Special Investigation, *Common Cause* 10, no. 4 (July/August 1984).

8. J. Turner, *The Aspartame/Nutrasweet Fiasco*, www.stevia.net/aspartame.htm.

9. Brackett and Waldron, *Sweet Misery: A Poisoned World*.

10. Ibid.

11. J. Bressler et al., "FDA Report on Searle," August 4, 1977, www.dorway.com/bressler.txt.

12. Gordon, "NutraSweet: Questions Swirl. Part 1: Did Searle Ignore Early Warning Signs?"

13. Preapproval, "Research & History of Aspartame," www.holisticmed.com/aspartame/history.faq.

14. A. Constantine, "History of Aspartame," 2004, www.wnho.net/history_of_aspartame.htm.

15. Brackett and Waldron, *Sweet Misery: A Poisoned World*.

16. Gordon, "NutraSweet: Questions Swirl, Part 1: Did Searle Ignore Early Warning Signs?"

17. Brackett and Waldron, *Sweet Misery: A Poisoned World*.

18. Constantine, "History of Aspartame."

19. U.S. General Accounting Office, "Briefing Report to the Honorable Howard Metzenbaum, U.S. Senate; Food and Drug Administraion, Six Former HHS Employees' Involvement In Aspartame's Approval," GAO/HRD-86-109BR, July 1986.

20. Food and Drug Administration, "Aspartame in Carbonated Beverages Approved," FDA Talk Paper, July 1, 1983.

21. Federal Register 48:31376, July 8, 1983.

22. F. Graves, "Results of *Common Cause* Magazine Investigation of FDA's Approval of Aspartame," July 1984.

23. "Morbidity and Mortality Weekly Report," www.cdc.gov.

24. R. Walton, "Survey of Aspartame Studies:Correlation of Outcome and Funding Sources," http://www.dorway.com/peerrev.html.

25. Paul M Ridker, MD, and Jose Torres, BA, "Reported Outcomes in Major Cardiovascular Clinical Trials Funded by For-Profit and Not-for-Profit Organizations: 2000-2005," *Journal of the American Medical Association* 295, no. 19 (May 17, 2006): 2270-74, http://cmsadmin.mercola.com/wkst/articleEdit.asp?http://jama.ama-assn.org/cgi/content/short/295/19/2270.

26. http://www.dorway.com/betty/review1.txt

27. J. Bressler, et al. "FDA Report on Searle" August 4, 1977. Available: dorway.com/bressler.txt.

28. "Is Neotame (Sweetener 2000) Safe?" www.alkalizeforhealth.net/Lsweetdebate26.htm.
29. "Monsanto Announces Sale of Sweetener Ingredient Business," http://www.monsanto.com/monsanto/layout/media/00/03-27-00.asp.
30. Anonymous food industry insider
31. Roberts, *Aspartame Disease: An Ignored Epidemic*.
32. Russell Blaylock, *Excitotoxins: The Taste That Kills*. MD Health Press (NM) 1996.
33. R. G. Walton, "Seizure and Mania after High Intake of Aspartame," *Psychosomatics* 27, no. 3 [March 1986]: 218, 220.
34. W. M. Pardridge, "The Safety of Aspartame," *Journal of the American Medical Association* 256, no. 19 (November 21, 1986): 267.
35. M. Warner, "The Lowdown on Sweet," *New York Times*, February 12, 2006, http://www.nytimes.com/2006/02/12/business/yourmoney/12sweet.html?pagewanted=1&ei=5088&en=f5f573accc334534&ex=1297400400&partner=rssnyt&emc=rss.
36. Jan Jensen. "Aspartame—The World's Best Ant Poison," *The Idaho Observer* (June 2006), http://www.proliberty.com/observer/20060612.htm. Reprinted with permission.
37. H. O. Adami, L. B. Signorello, and D. Trichopoulos, "Towards an Understanding of Breast Cancer Etiology," *Seminars in Cancer Biology* 8 (1998): 255–62.
38. O. M. Sejersted, D. Jacobsen, S. Ovrebo, and H. Jansen, "Formate Concentrations in Plasma from Patients Poisoned with Methanol," *Acta Medica Scandinavica* 213 (1983): 105–10.
39. J. Bowen, "Aspartame Toxicity and Methanol, Ethanol, Pectin, Methyl Alcohol," www.321recipes.com.
40. Woodrow Monte, "Report Aspartame: Methanol and the Public Health," *Journal of Applied Nutrition* 36, no. 1 (1984), http://www.dorway.com/monte84.html.
41. Brackett and Waldron, *Sweet Misery: A Poisoned World*.
42. Ibid.
43. R. J. Louis, *Sax's Dangerous Properties of Industrial Materials*, 8th ed. (New York: Van Nostrand Reinhold, 1992), 2251–52.
44. The Wysong E-Health Letter, www.wysong.net/health/hl_839.shtml.
45. R. J. Louis, *Sax's Dangerous Properties of Industrial Materials*, 8th ed. (New York: Van Nostrand Reinhold, 1992), 2251–52.
46. EPA official Web site, www.epa.gov.
47. G. R. Schwartz, "Aspartame and Breast and Other Cancers," *Western Journal of Medicine*, 1999, 300.
48. K. Marshall, *User's Guide to Protein and Amino Acids* (Laguna Beach, CA: Basic Health Publications, 2005).
49. Blaylock, *Excitotoxins: The Taste That Kills*.
50. J. W. Olney, L. G. Sharpe, and R. D. Feigin, "Glutamate Induced Brain Damage in Infant Primates," *Journal of Neuropathology and Experimental Neurology* 31 (1972): 464–88.
51. J. W. Olney, "Glutamate, a Neurotoxic Transmitter," *Journal of Child Neurology* 4 (1989): 218–26.

52. S. Fichtlscherer, S. Breuer, V. Schachinger, S. Dimmeler, and A. M. Zeiher, "C-Reactive Protein Levels Determine Systemic Nitric Oxide Bioavailability in Patients with Coronary Artery Disease," *European Heart Journal* 25, no. 16 (August 2004): 1412–18.

53. C. Napoli, V. Sica, F. de Nigris, O. Pignalosa, M. Condorelli, L. J. Ignarro, and A. Liguori, "Sulfhydryl Angiotensin—Converting Enzyme Inhibition Induces Sustained Reduction of Systemic Oxidative Stress and Improves the Nitric Oxide Pathway in Patients with Essential Hypertension," *American Heart Journal* 148, no. 1 (July 2004): e5.

54. H. J Roberts, *Aspartame Disease: An Ignored Epidemic,* (West Palm Beach: Sunshine Sentinel Press, 2001).

55. J. W. Olney, *Brain Research* 112: 420–24.

56. American Dietetic Association, "Use of Nutritive and Nonnutritive Sweeteners," http://www.eatright.org/cps/rde/xchg/ada/hs.xsl/advocacy_adap0598_ENU_HTML.htm.

57. "Safety of Amino Acids," Life Sciences Research Office, FASEB, FDA Contract no. 223-88-2124, Task Order no. 8.

58. G. R. Kerr and H. A. Waisman, *Transplacental Ratios of Serum-Free Amino Acids During Pregnancy in the Rhesus Monkey; Amino Acid Metabolism and Genetic Variation* (New York: McGraw Hill, 1967).

59. www.ncbi.nlm.nih.gov/entrez/query.fcgi.

60. S. K. Van den Eeden, T. D. Koespell, W. T. Longstreth et al., "Aspartame Ingestion and Headaches: A Randomized Crossover Trial," *Neurology* 44 (1994): 1787–93.

61. R. B. Lipton, L. C. Newman, J. Cohen, and S. Solomon, "Aspartame and Headache," *Neurology* 38 (1988): 356.

62. R. B. Lipton, L. C. Newman, J. S. Cohen, and S. Solomon, "Aspartame as a Dietary Trigger of Headaches," *Headaches* 23 (1989): 90–92.

63. S. M. Koehler and A. Glaros, "The Effect of Aspartame in Migraine Headache," *Headache* 28 (1988): 10–14.

64. J. W. Olney, N. B. Farber, E. Spitznagel, and L. N. Robbins, "Increasing Brain Tumor Rates: Is There a Link to Aspartame?" *Journal of Neuropathology and Experimental Neurology* 55 (1996): 1115–23.

65. Study E33-34 in Master File 134 on aspartame, on file at the FDA Hearing Clerk's Office 2001.

66. National Cancer Institute SEER Program Data, K. E. Jellinger et al., "Primary Central Nervous System Lymphomas: An Update," *Journal of the National Cancer Institute* 84 (1992): 414–22.

67. J. G. Gurney, J. M. Pogoda, and E. A. Holly, "Aspartame Consumption in Relation to Childhood Brain Tumor Risk: Results from a Case-Control Study," *Journal of the National Cancer Institute* 89 (1997): 1072–74.

68. M. Soffritti, F. Belpoggi, Degli, D. Esposti et al., "First Experimental Demonstration of the Multipotential Carcinogenic Effects of Aspartame Administered in the Feed to Sprague-Dawley Rats," *Environmental Health Perspectives* 114, no. 3 (March 2006): 379–85.

69. Jim Turner, "Delaney Lives! Reports of Delaney's death are greatly exaggerated." Available: wnho.net/delaney_lives.htm

70. 8/1/85 Senate, S 10839 – 10840.

71. R. G. Walton et al., "Adverse Reactions to Aspartame: Double-Blind Challenge in Patients from a Vulnerable Population," *Biology Psychiatry* 34 (1993): 13–17.

72. Ibid.

73. H. J. Roberts, "Neurological, Psychiatric, and Behavioral Reactions to Aspartame in 505 Aspartame Reactors," in R. J. Wurtman and E. R. Walker, eds., *Dietary Phenylalanine and Brain Function* (Boston: Birkhauser, 373–76.

74. The reference is the Study Design section of Dr. Walton's study: "NutraSweet Company denied the request from the authors to puchase aspartame. Therefore, analytically certified USP grade aspartame was purchased from Schweizerhall, Inc., Piscataway, NJ"; Ralph G. Walton et al., "Adverse Reactions to Aspartame: Double-Blind Challenge in Patients From a Vulnerable Population," *Biological Psychiatry* 34 (1993): 13-17.

75. R. J. Wurtman, press conference on Cable News Network (CNN), July 17, 1986.

76. U.S. Air Force, "Aspartame Alert," *Flying Safety* 48, no. 5 (May 1992): 20–21.

77. Ibid.

78. G. Martin-Amat, K. E. McMartin, S. S. Hayreh et al., "Methanol Poisoning: Ocular Toxicity Produced by Formate," *Toxicology and Applied Pharmacology* 45 (1978): 201–8.

79. Roberts, *Aspartame Disease: An Ignored Epidemic.*

80. W. L. Hall, D. J. Millward, P. J. Rogers, and L. M. Morgan, "Physiological Mechanisms Mediating Aspartame-Induced Satiety," *Physiology and Behavior* 78, nos. 4–5 (April 2003): 557–62.

81. L. N. Chen and E. S. Parham, "College Students' Use of High-Intensity Sweeteners Is Not Consistently Associated with Sugar Consumption," *Journal of the American Dietetic Association* 91 (1991): 686–90.

82. "U.S. Study Links Diet Pop to Obesity," June 15 2005, www.ctv.ca/servlet/ArticleNews/story/CTVNews/1118840585467_33/?hub=TopStories.

83. Betty Martini, "Interview with Dr. Roberts," 1998, www.dorway.com/hjrinv.txt.

84. Russell Blaylock, *Excitotoxins: The Taste That Kills* MD Health Press (NM) 1996.

85. C. Trocho et al., "Formaldehyde Accumulating from Aspartame Ingestion," 1998; "Formaldehyde Derived from Dietary Aspartame Binds to Tissue Components In Vitro," *Life Sciences* 63, no. 5 (1998): 337+; see study at: http://www.presidiotex.com/barcelona/.

86. References listed are available at the end of the following Web page: http://www.holisticmed.com/aspartame/scf2002-response.htm.

Other reviews on formaldehyde can be found at http://www.drthrasher.org/research.html

Shaham, J., Y. Bomstein, A. Meltzer, Z. Kaufman, E. Palma, J. Ribak, 1996. "DNA—protein Crosslinks, a Biomarker of Exposure to Formaldehyde—in vitro and in vivo Studies," Carcinogenesis, Volume 17, No. 1, page 121–125.

Main, D.M., T.J. Hogan, 1983. "Health Effect of Low-Level Exposure to Formaldehyde," Journal of Occupational Medicine, Volume 25, page 896-900.

Liu, Kai-Shen, et al., 1993. "Irritant Effects of Formaldehyde Exposure in Mobile Homes," Environmental Health Perspectives, Volume 94, page 91-94.

Wantke, F., C.M. Demmer, P. Tappler, M. Gotz, R. Jarisch, 1996. "Exposure to Gaseous Formaldehyde Induces IgE-Mediated Sensitization To Formaldehyde in School-Children," Clinical and Experimental Allergy, Volume 26, pages 276-280.

Srivastava, A.K., et al., 1992. "Clinical studies of employees in a sheet-forming process at a paper mill," Veterinary and Human Toxicology, Volume 34, No. 6, page 525–527.

Olsen, J.H., M. Dossing, 1982. "Formaldehyde induced symptoms in day care centers," American Industrial Hygeine Association Journal, Volume 43, Number 5, pages 366-370, 1982.

Burdach, S., K. Wechselberg, 1980. "Damages to health in schoos. Complaints caused by the use of formaldehyde-emitting materials in school buildings," Fortschritte Med, Volume 98, Number 11, pages 379-384, 1980.

Suruda, A., et al., 1993. "Cytogenic effects of formaldehyde exposure in students of mortuary science," Cancer Epidemiology and Biomarkers," Volume 2, Number 5, pages 453-460, 1993.

Taskinen, H.K., et al., 1999. "Reduced fertility among female wood workers exposed to formaldehyde," American Journal of Industrial Medicine, Volume 36, Number 1, pages 206-212, 1999.

Kilburn, K.H., 2000. "Indoor air effects after building renovation and in manufactured homes," American Journal of Medical Science, Volume 320, Number 4, pages 249-254, 2000.

Kilburn, K.H., 1994. "Neurobehavioral impairment and seizures from formaldehyde," Archives of Environmental Health, Volume 49, Number 1, pages 37-44, 1994.

Proietti, L., P.B. Sandona, B. Longo, S. Gulino, D. Duscio, 2002. "Occupational exposure to formaldehyde at a service of pathologic anatomy," Giornale Italiano di Medicina del Lavoro ed Ergonomia, Volume 24, Number 1, pages 32-34, 2002.

Maroziene, L., R. Grazuleviciene, 2002. "Maternal exposure to low-level aire pollution and pregnancy outcomes: a population-based study," Environmental Health, Volume 1, Number 1, page 6+, 2002.

Kilburn, K.H., B.C., Seidman, R. Warshaw, 1985. "Neurobehavioral and respiratory symptoms of formaldehyde and xylene exposure in histology technicians," Archives of Environmental Health, Volume 40, Number 4, pages 229-233, 1985.

87. Scorecard: The Pollution Information Web site, http://scorecard.org/env-releases/facility.tcl?tri_id=30903THNTR1750L#maps.

88. Ibid.

89. Brackett and Waldron, *Sweet Misery: A Poisoned World.*

90. "Aspartame and the FDA" (April 20, 1995) presidiotex.com/aspartame/Facts/Aspartame_and_the_FDA/aspartame_and_the_fda.html

91. H. Roberts, *Aspartame Disease: An Ignored Epidemic* (West Palm Beach: Sunshine Sentinel Press, Inc., 2001).

CHAPTER FOUR

1. Carney, Beth, "It's Not All Sweetness for Splenda," *Business Week* Online, http://www.businessweek.com/bwdaily/dnflash/jan2005/nf20050119_5391_db014.htm.

2. "The Secret Dangers of Splenda (Sucralose), an Artificial Sweetener," http://www.mercola.com/2000/dec/3/sucralose_dangers.htm.

3. Elizabeth Esfahani, "Finding the Sweet Spot," November 1, 2005, http://money.cnn.com/magazines/business2/business2_archive/2005/11/01/8362835/index.htm.

4. "FDA Approves New High-Intensity Sweetener Sucralose," http://www.fda.gov/bbs/topics/ANSWERS/ANS00859.html.

5. Stephen Fox, "Personal Perspective: New Era of Consumer Protection Possible, if Legislature Acts on Aspartame Ban," *New Mexican*, January 20, 2006, http://www.freenewmexican.com/news/38198.html.

6. "Holland Sweetener Drops Aspartame," FreeMarketNews.com, April 12, 2006, http://www.freemarketnews.com/WorldNews.asp?nid=11120.

7. Burkhard Bilger, "The Search for Sweet," *New Yorker*, May 22, 2006.

8. H. C. Grice and L. A. Goldsmith, "Sucralose—An Overview of the Toxicity Data," *Food and Chemical Toxicology* 38 (2000): S1–S6.

9. http://plaza.ufl.edu/mr2/MAN6636/splendaPaper.doc.

10. Melanie Warner, "US: Senomyx's Fake Flavors," *New York Times*, April 6, 2005, http://www.corpwatch.org/article.php?id=12053.

11. "Enhancing the Regulatory Decision-Making Approval Process for Direct Food Ingredient Technologies," Institute of Medicine (IOM), The National Academies Press, 1999, http://darwin.nap.edu/openbook/0309064864/html/105.html.

12. "Formal Comment Period on Food Additive Petitions Requested," *Food Chemistry News*, July 6, 1992, 36–37.

13. Anonymous source

14. Interview with two food industry insiders who wish to remain anonymous.

15. Interview with two food industry insiders who wish to remain anonymous.

16. Bilger, "The Search for Sweet."

17. www.SweetDeception.com/Patent; the Chemical Abstracts Service Registry number for sucralose: 56038-13-2, http://www.cas.org/.

18. http://72.14.203.104/search?q=cache:y1d0M1v-vksJ:www.ehs.psu.edu/hazmat/highly_hazardous_chemicals.pdf+chlorine+class+one+carcinogen+osha&hl=en&gl=us&ct=clnk&cd=1&client=firefox-a.

19. "Poison Gases," http://www.spartacus.schoolnet.co.uk/FWWgas.htm.

20. Deanna Lewis and Ron Chepesiuk, "The Chlorine Debate: A Selected Bibliography," April 1995, http://egj.lib.uidaho.edu/egj03/lewis01.html.

21. "Frequently Asked Questions about SPLENDA® Brand Sweetener," http://www.splenda.com/page.jhtml;jsessionid=XRM3VEYLBAF24CQPCB3SUYYKB2IIWNSC?id=splenda/faqs/nocalorie.inc#q2.

22. http://www.eurochlor.org/nature.

23. Anthony Carpi, "Chemical Bonding," http://www.visionlearning.com/library/module_viewer.php?mid=55.

24. Leo Morin, PhD, "The Art and Science of Aquarium Management," Seachem.com, http://www.seachem.com/support/Articles/Art_Science.html.

25. James Bowen, "The Lethal Science of Splenda, A Poisonous Chlorocarbon," May 2005, www.wnho.net/splenda_chlorocarbon.htm.

26. Kevin Ban, "Toxicity, Hydrocarbon Insecticides," emedicine.com, December 2005, http://www.emedicine.com/emerg/topic255.htm.

27. Ibid.

28. R. Carson, *Silent Spring* (New York: Mariner Books, 2002).

29. Kevin Ban, "Toxicity, Hydrocarbon Insecticides," emedicine.com, December 2005, http://www.emedicine.com/emerg/topic255.htm.

30. Christine Miller (Patterson, Belknap, Webb & Tyler) to Joseph Mercola, letter, "Web Site Statements Regarding Sucralose," September 28, 2004, 5.

31. "Dicofol," *Pesticide News*, http://www.pan-uk.org/pestnews/actives/dicofol.htm.

32. ToxFAQs™ for Methoxychlor, http://www.atsdr.cdc.gov/tfacts47.html.

33. http://pmep.cce.cornell.edu/profiles/extoxnet/carbaryl-dicrotophos/chlorobenzilate-ext.html.

34. http://www.atsdr.cdc.gov/tfacts31.html.

35. http://www.atsdr.cdc.gov/tfacts12.html.

36. Extension Toxicology Network, http://extoxnet.orst.edu/pips/pentachl.htm.

37. http://greenpeace.org.au/toxics/pops/hcb.html.

38. http://www.greenfacts.org/dioxins/dioxins.htm#4.

39. Michael Belliveau and Stephen Lester, "PVCs Bad News Comes in 3s," http://www.besafenet.com/pvc/pvcreports.htm.

40. "ToxFAQs™ for 1,2-Dichloroethane," September 2001, http://www.atsdr.cdc.gov/tfacts38.html.

41. "ToxFAQs™ for 1,1,1-Trichloroethane," September 2004, http://www.atsdr.cdc.gov/tfacts38.html.

42. For all entries except those listed: http://www.fws.gov/pacific/ecoservices/envicon/pim/reports/contaminantinfo/contaminants.html.

43. Michael Jacobson, "Splenda Should Stop Confusing Customers, Says CSPI," February 2005, www.cspinet.org.

44. "Dieticians Think Splenda Ads Are 'RottenJ&J/McNeil's Splenda Ads Win Canadian 'Rotten Apple' Prize," PR Newswire, March 2005, http://sev.prnewswire.com/food-beverages/20050325/DCTH02324032005-1.html.

45. Colette Bouchez, "Dieticians Say Splenda Is Not the Same as Sugar," WebMD, February 2005, http://www.webmd.com/content/article/100/105877.htm.

46. "FDA Final Rule for Sucralose Approval," http://www.cfsan.fda.gov/~lrd/fr980403.html. Section 102.5(a) is listed in appendix G.

47. "Sucralose," http://www.wholefoodsmarket.com/healthinfo/sucralose.html.

48. Lorraine Heller, "US Sugar Industry Wins Round Against Splenda," Confectionary

News.com, March 2006, http://www.confectionerynews.com/news/ng.asp?n=66826 -mcneil-nutritionals-sugar-association-splenda.

49. "US sugar industry wins round against Splenda" Available: foodnavigator-usa.com/ news-by-product/news.asp?id=66826&idCat=88&k=us-sugar-industry

50. "Consumer Organizations Ask Attorney General to Review Splenda's Advertising Practices," September 23, 2005, www.prnewswire.com/cgi-bin/stories.pl?ACCT= 109&STORY=/www/story/09-23-2005/0004114301&EDATE.

51. 21 CFR Part 172 [Docket NO. 87F-0086 Food Additives Permitted for Direct Addition to Food for Human Consumptions; Sucralose]. Study E051.

52. S. W. Mann, M. M. Yuschak, S. J. Amyes et al., "A Carcinogenicity Study of Sucralose in the CD-1 Mouse," *Food and Chemical Toxicology* 38, suppl. 2 (2000): S91-7.

53. http://www.mercola.com/2000/dec/3/sucralose_testimonials.htm.

54. N. H. Mezitis, C. A. Maggio, P. Koch et al., "All Glycemic Effect of a Single High Oral Dose of the Novel Sweetener Sucralose in Patients with Diabetes," *Diabetes Care* 19, no. 9 (September 1996): 1004–5; N. Y. Reyna, C. Cano, V. J. Bermudez et al., "Sweeteners and Beta-glucans Improve Metabolic and Anthropometrics Variables in Well-Controlled Type 2 Diabetic Patients," *American Journal of Therapeutics* 10, no. 6 (November–December 2003): 438-43.

55. "The Lowdown on Sweets," *New York Times*, February 12, 2006, http://www.nytimes. com/2006/02/12/business/yourmoney/12sweet.html?pagewanted=3&ei=5088&en= f5f573accc334534&ex=1297400400&partner=rssnyt&emc=rss.

56. Memorandum, William L. Roth, PhD, Pharmacologist, HFS-506 Subject Review of Metabolic and Pharmacokinetic Studies (E163 and E164) on Sucralose (TGS): FAP 7A3987 (McNeil Specialty Products Co.) to Blondell Anderson, Division of Product Policy, HFS-207, October 26, 1994.

57. The Potential Dangers of Sucralose: Reader Testimonials, http://www.mercola.com/ 2000/dec/3/sucralose_testimonials.htm.

58. "The Science of Splenda Brand Sweetener (Sucralose)," www.Splenda.com, http:// www.splendaprofessional.com/page.jhtml?id=/splendaprofessional/include/ science.inc.

59. FDA Final Rule, Federal Register 63, no. 64 (April 3, 1998), www.cfsan.fda.gov/ ~lrd/fr980403.html.

60. B. A. John, S. G. Wood, and D. R. Hawkins, "The Pharmacokinetics and Metabolism of Sucralose in the Mouse," *Food and Chemical Toxicology* 38 (2000): S107-S110.

61. FDA Final Rule, Federal Register 63, no. 64 (April 3, 1998), www.cfsan.fda.gov/ ~lrd/fr980403.html.

62. A. Roberts, A. G. Renwick, J. Sims, and D. J. Snodin, "Sucralose Metabolism and Pharmacokinetics in Man," *Food and Chemical Toxicology* 38 (2000): S31-S41.

63. A. D. Anderson, P. K. Jain, S. Fleming, P. Poon, C. J. Mitchell, and J. MacFie, "Evaluation of a Triple Sugar Test of Colonic Permeability in Humans," *Acta Physiologica Scandinavica* 2, no. 182 (2004): 171–77.

64. "The Science of Splenda Brand Sweetener (Sucralose)," www.Splenda.com, http://www. splendaprofessional.com/page.jhtml?id=/splendaprofessional/include/science.inc.

NOTES

65. http://www.ffcr.or.jp/zaidan/FFCRHOME.nsf/pages/e-kousei-sucra.
66. http://www.humpath.com/article.php3?id_article=4672.
67. William Roth, PhD, Pharmacologist to Review Staff, Office of Pre-Market Approval, Department of Health & Human Services. Memorandum, 26 October 1994, Subject: Summary of Sucralose Pharmacokinetic Studies To-Date, 4.
68. "The Science of Splenda® Brand Sweetener (Sucralose)," www.Splenda.com, emphasis added.
69. B. A. John, S. G. Wood, and D. R. Hawkins, "The Pharmacokinetics and Metabolism of Sucralose in the Rabbit,"
Food and Chemical Toxicology 38, suppl. 2 (2000): S111±S113.
70. McNeil Specialty Products Food Additive Petition 7A3987, (1987) (Sucralose) and enlarged colons.
71. "Sucralose: A Scientific and Safety Review," 10, www.Splenda.com, www.splendaprofessional.com/page.jhtml?id=/splendaprofessional/include/science.inc, emphasis added.
72. B. A. John, S. G. Wood, and D. R. Hawkins, "The Pharmacokinetics and Metabolism of Sucralose in the Rabbit," Food and Chemical Toxicology 38, suppl. 2 (2000): S111±S113.
73. Dr. John Modderman of the Food Color and Additives Review Section, memo.
74. "The Science of Splenda Brand Sweetener (Sucralose)," www.Splenda.com, http://www.splendaprofessional.com/page.jhtml?id=/splendaprofessional/include/science.inc.
75. Stuart Graham, Additives Evaluation Branch (H FF-158), Department of Health & Human Services To Ms. Blondell Anderson Through: G.N. Biddle, PhD, Memorandum, 8 August 1991, Subject: Sucralose—Final Review and Evaluation FOOD ADDITIVE PETITION NO. 7A3987, Washington, D.C., 21.
76. A. Coghlan, "Shrunken Thymus Glands Spark Sweetener Controversy," New Scientist, 1991, 1796.
77. J. P. Finn and G. H. Lord, "Neurotoxicity Studies on Sucralose and Its Hydrolysis Products with Special Reference to Histopathologic and Ultrastructural Changes," Food and Chemical Toxicology 38, suppl. 2 (2000): S7±S17.
78. W. C. Ford and G. M. Waites, "A Reversible Contraceptive Action of Some 6-chloro-deoxy Sugars in the Male Rat," Journal of Reproduction and Fertility 52 (1978): 153–57.
79. Ibid.
80. Stuart Graham, Additives Evaluation Branch (H FF-158), Department of Health & Human Services To Ms. Blondell Anderson Through: G.N. Biddle, PhD, Memorandum, 8 August 1991, Subject: Sucralose—Final Review and Evaluation FOOD ADDITIVE PETITION NO. 7A3987, Washington, D.C., 21; studies cited: E085.
81. Studies cited:
   "1,6-dichloro-1, 6-dideoxyfructose: Investigation of Effects on Bone Marrow Chromosomes of the Rat after

Acute and Subacute Oral Administration," EO19.

"1,6–dichloro-l ,6-dideoxyfructose: Assessment of Its Mutagenic Potential in Histidine Auxotrophs of Salmonella typhimurium," E020.

"1 ,6-dichloro-l ,6-dideoxyfructose: Assessment of Its Mutagenic Potential in Drosophila melanoqaster, Using the Sex-Linked Recessive Lethal Test," E021.

"Evaluation of Test Article 1,6-dichlorofructose (MRI #536) for Mutagenic Potential Employing the L5178Y TK+/ Mutagenesis Assay," E022.

"Salmonella/Mammalian Microsome Plate Incorporation Mutagenesis Assay," E023.

"Evaluation of Test Article 1, 6-dichlorofructose (MRI #629) for Mutagenic Potential EmDloying the L5178Y TK+/ Mutagenesis Assay," E024.

82–85. FDA studies labeled as E148, E054, E052, E032, E053.

86. Ford and Waites, *Journal of Reproduction and Fertility* 65:177–83.

87. E116, emphasis added.

88. James Griffiths, Division of Toxicology, Additives Evaluation Branch, Department of Health & Human Services to Direct Additives Branch/Blonell Anderson, Memorandum, 22 August 1988, Subject: Review of Sucralose Metabolism and Pharmacokinetics Studies. Food Additive Petition 7A3987, Washington, D.C., 10, emphasis added.

89. 1,6-Dichloro-1,6-dideoxyfructose: Metabolism in the Rat. Study E147. Laboratory: Department of Biochemistry, University College, Wales, UK, March 8, 1988, File location: FAP 7A3987, vol. 98, A002598-02661.

90. A. Roberts, Renwick, A. G., Sims, J., and Snodin, D. J., "Sucralose Metabolism and Pharmacokinetics in Man," *Food Chem Toxicol* 38 (2000): S31-S41

91. FDA Final Rule. Federal Register: April 3, 1998 (Volume 63, Number 64) Available: cfsan.fda.gov/~lrd/fr980403.html

92. James Bowen, "The Lethal Science of Splenda, A Poisonous Chlorocarbon," May 8, 2005, http://www.wnho.net/splenda_chlorocarbon.htm.

93. "The Science of Splenda Brand Sweetener (Sucralose)," www.Splenda.com, http://www.splendaprofessional.com/page.jhtml?id=/splendaprofessional/include/science.inc.

94. Ibid.

95. 1,6-dichloro-1,6-dideoxy-, -D-fructofuranosyl-4-choro-4-deoxy- ·-D-galactopyranoside (TGS): Absorption, Tissue Distribution and Excretion in the Rat.

96. William Roth, PhD, Pharmacologist to Review Staff, Office of Pre-Market Approval, Department of Health & Human Services. Memorandum, 26 October 1994, Subject: Summary of Sucralose Pharmacokinetic Studies To-Date, 4, emphasis added.

97. "Sucralose: A Scientific and Safety Review," 10, www.Splenda.com, www.splendaprofessional.com/page.jhtml?id=/splendaprofessional/include/science.inc.

98. FDA Memorandum from G. Biddle to B. Anderson. (August 8, 1990) pg. 2 Regarding 1. 1 ,6-dichloro-l ,6-dideoxy-B-il-fructofuranosyl-4-chl oro-4-deoxy—D galactopyranoslde (TGS): Absorption, Tissue Distribution And Excretion In The Rat. EO04.

99. J. Kille, J. Tesh et al., "Sucralose: Assessment of Teratogenic Potential in the Rat and the Rabbit," *Food and Chemical Toxicology* 38, supp. 2 (2002): S43-52.

100. FDA Final Rule, Federal Register 63, no. 64 (April 3, 1998), E056, E032, www.cfsan.fda.gov/~lrd/fr980403.html.

101. Jennifer Bogo, "Children at Risk: Widespread Chemical Exposure Threatens Our Most Vulnerable Population," Emagazine.com Xii, no. 5 (September/October 2001), www.emagazine.com/view/?1074.

102. Susan Resinick, "Warning: A Beautiful Lawn Could Be Hazardous to Your Child's Health," Projo.com, March 2003, www.projo.com/health/content/projo_20030330_pestx.1602d.html.

103. FDA Final Rule, Federal Register 63, no. 64 (April 3, 1998), www.cfsan.fda.gov/~lrd/fr980403.html.

104. Y. Sasaki, S. Kawaguchi et al., "The Comet Assay with 8 Mouse Organs: Results with 39 Currently Used Food Additives," *Mutation Research* 519, nos. 1–2 (August 26, 2002): 103–19.

105. E004.

106. FDA Final Rule. Federal Register: April 3, 1998 (Volume 63, Number 64) Available: cfsan.fda.gov/~lrd/fr980403.html and Malkins Legal Firm To: FDA. Letter. September 27, 1999. Re: Sucralose

107. FDA Final Rule, Federal Register 63, no. 64 (April 3, 1998), www.cfsan.fda.gov/~lrd/fr980403.html.

108. Mann, S. W., Yuschak, M. M., Amyes, S. J., et al, "A carcinogenicity study of sucralose in the CD-1 mouse," *Food Chem Toxicol*, 2000;38 Suppl 2:S91-7.

109. Mann, S., Yuschak, M., et al, "A Combined Chronic Toxicity/Carcinogenicity Study of Sucralose in Sprague-Dawley Rats," *Food and Chemical Toxicology* 38 (Suppl. 2) (2000) S71-S89.

110. FDA Final Rule for Sucralose http://www.cfsan.fda.gov/~lrd/fr980403.html

111. Ibid

112. Ibid

113. Ibid.

114. A. Coghlan, "Shrunken Thymus Glands Spark Sweetener Controversy," *New Scientist*, 1991, 1796.

115. FDA Final Rule for Sucralose.

116. Ibid.

117. Ibid

118. The Potential Dangers of Sucralose: Reader Testimonials, http://www.mercola.com/2000/dec/3/sucralose_testimonials.htm.

119. FDA, "A Food Labeling Guide—Appendix A: Definitions of Nutrient Content Claims," http://www.cfsan.fda.gov/~dms/flg-6a.html.

120. Richard Bernstein, *Dr. Bernstein's Diabetes Solution* (Boston: Little, Brown and Company, 2003), 138, emphasis added.

121. "Sucralose: An Excellent Safety Profile for All Your Patients," www.Splenda.com, http://www.splendaprofessional.com/page.jhtml;jsessionid=L5K25DEWK

TYNICQPCCECUYYKB2IIWNSC?id=/splendaprofessional/include/safety_
profile.inc.

122. H. Grice and L. Goldsmith, "Sucralose—An Overview of the Toxicity Data," *Food and Chemical Toxicology* 38, suppl. 2 (2000): S1±S6.

123. C. Ness, "Splenda 101," *San Francisco Chronicle*, September 15, 2004, http://www.sfgate.com/cgi-bin/article.cgi?f=/chronicle/archive/2004/09/15/FDGA58M7L21.DTL.

124. Nancy Stohs, "Substitute May Not Be Sweetest Solution," MilwaukeeMarketplace.com, November 2004, http://www.milwaukeemarketplace.com/story/index.aspx?id=273596.

125. Scorecard.org. Available: scorecard.org/env-releases/facility.tcl?tri_id=36553 MCNLSINDUS#major_chemical_releases

126. "Sucralose Plant Neighbors in South Alabama Sue over Noise, Odor," www.WPMI.com, June 2006, http://www.wpmi.com/news/local/story.aspx?content_id=E520ED84-1364-40E5-AD8A-A80AE1A30802.

127. Bill Finch, "Crowd Packs Church During Permit Hearing," ALAEAVs, April 27, 2005, http://www.alaleavs.org/shownews.asp?newsid=1027.

128. "Tate & Lyle to Build New Sucralose Plant in Singapore," November 2004, http://193.35.126.50/PressReleases/PressRelease1287.asp.

129. Jacobson, Michael. "Splenda Should Stop Confusing Consumers, Says CSPI" *CSPI Newsroom*. Available: cspinet.org/new/200502141.html

ADDITIONAL CHAPTER FOUR REFERENCES

"Splenda Sickness," April 2005, splendasickness.blogspot.com.
"Sucralose Partners Prepare for New Challenges," February 2004, foodnavigator.com.

CHAPTER FIVE

1. Mannette Loudon, "Prescription Drug Alert: Millions at Risk fromPossibly Deadly Side Effects," *Crusador* 25 (June/July 2005), http://www.mercola.com/2005/aug/13/secrets_of_the_fda_revealed_by_top_insider_doctor.htm.

2. *Timothy D. Warner, Francesco Giuliano, Ivana Vojnovic et al.,* "Nonsteroid Drug Selectivities for Cyclo-oxygenase-1 Rather Than Cyclo-oxygenase-2 Are Associated with Human Gastrointestinal Toxicity: A Full In Vitro Analysis," *Proceedings of the National Academy of Sciences of the United States of America* 96, no. 13 (June 22, 1999): 7563-68, http://www.pnas.org/cgi/content/full/96/13/7563.

3. Joseph Mercola. "New Painkiller Might Be A Bitter Pill For Some Patients." http://www.mercola.com/1999/archive/painkiller.htm >.

4. John Robbins. *Diet for a New America: How Your Food Choices Affect Your Health, Happiness and the Future of Life on Earth* (H J Kramer Inc. and New World Library:Tiburon 1987)

5. Andy Rowell, "Welcome to Wal-World," *Multinational Monitor*, October 2003, http://www.projectcensored.org/publications/2005/25.html.

6. [author?]"Competing With Wal-Mart" (June 5, 2004) at: livelydebate.com/archives/category/food/

7. "Wal-Mart Eyes Organic Foods," *New York Times*, May 12, 2006, http:// select.nytimes. com/gst/abstract.html?res=F50A15FE3F5A0C718DDDAC0894DE404482.

8. Michael Pollan, "Mass Natural," *New York Times*, June 2006, http://www.nytimes.com/2006/06/04/magazine/04wwln_lede.html?ex=1307073600&en=07310c42ac1a390c&ei=5088&partner=rssnyt&emc=rss.

9. R. Doll, "Chronic and Degenerative Disease: Major Causes of Morbidity and Death," *American Journal of Clinical Nutrition* 62 (1995): 1301S-1305S, http://www.ajcn.org/cgi/reprint/62/6/1301S.

10. American Cancer Society 2005 Annual Report, http://www.cancer.org/downloads/AA/AnnualReport_2005.pdf.

11. C. Cowie, K. F. Rust, D. D. Byrd-Holt et al., "Prevalence of Diabetes and Impaired Fasting Glucose in Adults in the U.S. Population," National Health and Nutrition Examination Survey 1999–2002, *Diabetes Care* 29 (June 2006): 1263–68.

12. D. A. Bennett, MD, J. A. Schneider, MD, J. L. Bienias et al., "Mild Cognitive Impairment Is Related to Alzheimer Disease Pathology and Cerebral Infarctions," *Neurology* 64 (2005): 834-8411, http://www.neurology.org/cgi/content/abstract/64/5/834?maxto show=&HITS=10&hits=10&RESULTFORMAT=&fulltext=bennett&searchid=11111 66148606_3968&stored_search=&FIRSTINDEX=0&volume=64&issue=5&journal code=neurology>.

13. http://www.monsanto.com/monsanto/layout/about_us/timeline/default.asp.

14. http://www.jnj.com/product/categories/Nutritionals.htm.

15. David Barboza, "As Biotech Crops Multiply Consumers Get Little Choice," *New York Times*, June 10, 2001, http://www.nytimes.com/2001/06/10/business/10GENE.html? ex=1146456000&en=8e80be37a8fa2f5c&ei=5070 >.

16. A. E. Gallo, "Food Advertising in the United States," in E. Frazao, ed., *American's Eating Habits: Changes & Consequences* (Washington, D.C.: USDA, 1999), 173–80.

17. M. Nestle, *Food Politics: How the Food Industry Influences Nutrition and Health* (University of California Press, Berkeley 2002).

18. Ibid.

19. S. Fried, *Bitter Pills: Inside the Hazardous World of Legal Drugs* (New York: Bantam, 1998).

20. FDA Talk Paper T97-6, January 30, 1997, http://www.fda.gov/bbs/topics/ANSWERS/ANS00783.html.

21. David Graham, "Testimony of David J. Graham" (November 18, 2004) at: Mercola.com/2005/mar/2/david_graham_testimonial.htm

22. Marcia Angell, *The Truth About Drug Companies* (New York: Random House, 2004), 209.

23. M. Adams, "If the Auto Industry Operated like Big Pharma: Fifteen Things You Might Notice." News Target, July 2005. At: newstarget.com.

24. Vera Sharay, "Pfizer Admits Guilt in Promotion of Neurotoxin—Agrees to Pay $430 Million" (May 16, 2004) Available: ahrp.org/infomail/04/05/16.php.

25. John Robbins, *May All Be Fed: Diet for a New World* (New York: Avon Books, 1992).

26. "The Formula Pushers—Infant Foods Multinationals Breaking the Rules," *Action for Corporate Accountability* 9 (1990): 3.

27. "Action Update," *Action for Corporate Accountability* Fall 1991, 1.
28. "Monsanto's Toxic Roundup," http://www.holisticmed.com/ge/roundup.html.
29. Organic Consumers Organization, "Protestors Destroy Two Plots of Genetically Engineered Corn in California," press release, July 28, 1999, http://www.organic consumers.org/ge/cagedestroy.cfm.
30. Organic Consumers Association, "Millions Against Monsanto," http://www.pure food.org/monlink.html.
31. C. Jenkins, "Criminal Investigation of Monsanto Corporation: Cover-Up of Dioxin Contamination in Products, Falsification of Dioxin Health Studies," November 1990, http://www.mindfully.org/Pesticide/Monsanto-Coverup-Dioxin-USEPA15 nov90.htm.
32. Ibid.
33. B. C. Martinson, M. S. Anderson, and R. de Vries, "Scientists Behaving Badly," *Nature* 435 (2005): 737–38.
34. S. Rampton and J. Stauber, *Trust Us, We're Experts!* (New York: Penguin Putnam, Inc., 2001).
35. Ibid.
36. Calorie Control Council, "Sucralose and Splenda® Brand Sweetener Offer Safe Options for Controlling Calories," www.caloriecontrol.org.
37. Nestle, *Food Politics*.
38. "American Council on Science and Health (ACSH)—Whose Interest Does It Serve?" Mindfully.org, http://www.mindfully.org/Pesticide/ACSH-Koop.htm.
39. Ibid.
40. Ibid.
41. "Diabetes Association Defends Cadbury Schweppes Deal," *Corporate Crime Reporter* 9, no. 20 (May 16, 2005), www.corporatecrimereporter.com.
42. American Dietetic Association, "Straight Answers about Aspartame," http://www. eatright.org/cps/rde/xchg/ada/hs.xsl/nutrition_1030_ENU_HTML.htm.
43. J. Drinkard, "Drugmakers Go Furthest to Sway Congress," *USA Today,* April 25, 2005, http://www.usatoday.com/money/industries/health/drugs/2005-04-25-drug-lobby-cover_x.htm.
44. Ibid.
45. M. Nestle, "Food Company Sponsorship of Nutrition Research and Professional Activities: a Conflict of Interest?" *Public Health Nutrition* 5, no. 4 (2001): 1015–22.
46. Nestle, *Food Politics: How the Food Industry Influences Nutrition and Health.*

ADDITIONAL CHAPTER FIVE REFERENCES

Brownell, K. D. *Food Fight: The Inside Story of the Food Industry, America's Obesity Crisis, and What We Can Do About It.* New York: McGraw-Hill, 2004.
Cohen, J. S. *Over Dose: The Case Against the Drug Companies.* New York: Penguin Putnam, Inc, 2001.
Greider, K. *The Big Fix: How the Pharmaceutical Industry Rips Off American Consumers.* New York: Public Affairs, 2003.

Stitt, P. A. *Beating the Food Giants*. Manitowoc, WI: Natural Press, 2003.

Strand, R. *Death by Prescription: The Shocking Truth Behind an Overmedicated Nation*. Nashville: Thomas Nelson Publishers, 2003.

Watson, J. L. *The Culture Politics of Food and Eating*. Malden, MA: Blackwell Publishing, 2005.

CHAPTER SIX

1. John Henkel, "Sugar Substitutes: Americans Opt for Sweetness and Lite," *FDA Consumer*, November–December 1999, rev. December 2004.

2. M. R. Weihrauch and V. Diehl, "Artificial sweeteners—Do They Bear a Carcinogenic Risk?" *Annals of Oncology* 10, no. 15 (2004): 1460–65.

3. R. Goldberg, "FDA Needs a Dose of Reform," *Wall Street Journal* (September 30, 2002): Sect A, 16.

4. A. V. Krebs, "Bitter Medicine," www.populist.com, 2002.

5. Interview with Dr. David Graham, senior FDA official for monitoring Vioxx toxicity, http://www.mercola.com/2005/aug/30/secrets_of_the_fda_revealed_by_top_insider_doctor_part_3.htm.

6. Gary Null, PhD, Carolyn Dean, MD, ND, Martin Feldman, MD, Debora Rasio, MD, and Dorothy Smith, PhD, "Modern Health Care System Is the Leading Cause of Death, Part I," Mercola.com, http://www.mercola.com/2004/jul/7/healthcare_death.htm.

7. David Willman, "How a New Policy Led to Seven Deadly Drugs" *LA Times* (Dec.20, 2000) at: biopsychiatry.com/bigpharma/fda.htm

8. C. Adams, "FDA Looks to Cure Its High Attrition Rate," *Wall Street Journal*, August 19, 2002, www.wsj.com.

9. Ibid.

10. Ibid.

11. "FDA Scientists Report Their Safety Concerns in Poll," *LA Times* July 21, 2006.

12. Diana Zuckerman, "FDA Reforms Without Industry Pressures," LA Times.com, May 6, 2006, http://www.latimes.com/news/opinion/letters/la-le-saturday6.1may06,0,2525215.story?coll=la-news-comment-letters.

13. Dennis Cauchon, FDA advisor with ties to the industry.

14. CSPI, "Conflicts of Interest on COX-2 Panel," www.cspinet.org.

15. FDA, "Statement by Linda A. Suydam, D.P.A., Senior Associate Commissioner, Food and Drug Administration Department of Health and Human Services, Before the Committee on Government Reform, U.S. House of Representatives," June 14, 2000, www.fda.gov.

16. "Investigational New Drug (IND) Application Process," http://www.fda.gov/cder/regulatory/applications/ind_page_1.htm.

17. Testimony of David J. Graham, MD, MPH, November 18, 2004, www.mercola.com/2005/mar/2/david_graham_testimonial.htm.

18. Ibid.

19. A. Black, "New England Journal of Medicine Accuses Merck of Deleting Important Vioxx Information from Study," February 15, 2006, http://www.newstarget.com/017875.html.

20. Testimony of David J. Graham, MD, MPH, November 18, 2004.
21. "Vioxx Verdict" at: slackdavis.com/newsletter_article.php/newsletter_article_id/argval/108/argname/back_link/argval/newsletters
22. A. Mathews and B. Martinez, "Warning Signs: E-Mails Suggest Merck Knew Vioxx's Dangers at Early Stage," *Wall Street Journal*, November 1, 2004.
23. "Report: Merck Knew of Vioxx Dangers Early," 2004, http://www.healthcentral.com/newsdetail/408/1505142.html.
24. Testimony of David J. Graham, MD, MPH, November 18, 2004.
25. L. Manette, "Prescription Drug Alert: Millions at Risk from Serious and Possibly Deadly Side Effects," *Crusador* 25 (June/July 2005).
26. "Correction to Cardiovascular Events Associated with Rofecoxib in a Colorectal Adenoma Chemoprevention," Trial *New England Journal of Medicine*, June 27, 2006.
27. Y. H. Hsu, J. C. Liu, P. F. Kao, C. N. Lee, Y. J. Chen, M. H. Hsieh, and P. Chan, "Antihypertensive Effect of Stevioside in Different Strains of Hypertensive Rats," *Zhonghua Yi Xue Za Zhi* 1, no. 65 (January 2002): 1–6.
28. D. Mozaffarian, M. B. Katan, A. Ascherio, M. J. Stampfer, and W. C. Willett, "Trans Fatty Acids and Cardiovascular Disease," *New England Journal of Medicine* 354, no. 15 (April 13, 2006): 1601–13.
29. Mary Enig and Sally Fallon, *Eat Fat, Lose Fat* (Penguin Group. New York 2005).

ADDITIONAL CHAPTER SIX REFERENCES
FDA Backgrounder, www.cfsan.fda.gov.
Higgs, R. *Hazards to Our Health? FDA Regulation of Health Care Products*. Oakland, CA.: The Independent Institute, 1995.
Hilts, P. J. *Protecting America's Health. The FDA, Business, and One Hundred Years of Regulation*. New York: Random House, Inc., 2003.
Lipsky, M. S., and L. K. Sharp. "From Idea to Market: The Drug Approval Process." *Journal of the American Board of Family Practice* 14 (2001): 362–67.
Prey, W. S. *A History of Nonprescription Product Regulation*. Binghamton, NY: Haworth Pr. Inc., 2003.

CHAPTER SEVEN
1. L. Manette, "Prescription Drug Alert: Millions at Risk from Serious and Possibly Deadly Side Effects," *Crusador* 25 (June/July 2005).

CHAPTER EIGHT
1. L. Bonvie, B. Bonvie, B., and D. Gates, *The Stevia Story* (CITY: B.E.D. Publications Co., 1997).
2. R. Curi, M. Alvarez, R. B. Bazotte, L. M. Botion, J. L. Goday, and A. Bracht, "Effect of Stevia Rebaudiana on Glucose Tolerance in Normal Adult Humans," *Brazilian Journal of Medical and Biological Research* 6, no. 19 (1986): 771–74.
3. H. Fujita and E. Tomoyoshi, "Safety and Utilization of Stevia Sweetener," *Shokumin Kogyo* 20, no. 22 (1979): 65–72.

4. Bonvie, Bonvie, and Gates, *The Stevia Story.*

5. Curi et al., "Effect of Stevia Rebaudiana on Glucose Tolerance in Normal Adult Humans."

6. M. H Hsieh, P. Chan, Y. M. Sue, J. C. Liu, T. H. Liang, T. Y. Huang, B. Tomlinson, M. S. Chow, P. F. Kao, and Y. J. Chen, "Efficacy and Tolerability of Oral Stevioside in Patients with Mild Essential Hypertension: A Two-Year, Randomized, Placebo-Controlled Study," *Clinical Therapeutics* 11 (November 25, 2003): 2797–808.

7. Y. H. Hsu, J. C. Liu, P. F. Kao, C. N. Lee, Y. J. Chen, M. H. Hsieh, and P. Chan, "Antihypertensive Effect of Stevioside in Different Strains of Hypertensive Rats," *Zhonghua Yi Xue Za Zhi* 1, no. 65 (January 2002): 1–6.

8. D. Richard, *Stevia Rebaudiana: Nature's Sweet Secret* (CITY: Vital Health Publishing, 1996).

9. Fujita and Tomoyoshi, "Safety and Utilization of Stevia Sweetener."

10. M. S. Melis, "Effects of Chronic Administration of Stevia Rebaudiana on Fertility in Rats," *Journal of Ethnopharmacology* 1. 2, no. 67 (November 1999): 157–61.

11. L. H. Lin, L. W. Lee, S. Y. Sheu, and P. Y. Lin, "Study on the Stevioside Analogues of Steviolbioside, Steviol, and Isosteviol 19-Alkyl Amide Dimers: Synthesis and Cytotoxic and Antibacterial Activity," *Chemical and Pharmaceutical Bulletin* 9, no. 52 (September 2004): 1117–22.

12. "Stevia Safety Information," www.dic.co.jp.

13. "Stevia Research and Studies," www.steviacanada.com.

14. "Cooking with Honey," www.kohala.net.

15. H. A. L. Wahdan, "Causes of the Antimicrobial Activity of Honey," *Infection* 26 (1998): 30–35

16. S. Kajiwara, H. Gandhi, and Z. Ustunol, "Effect of Honey on the Growth of and Acid Production by Human Intestinal Bifidobacterium Spp.: An In Vitro Comparison with Commercial Oligosaccharides and Inulin," *Journal of Food Protection* 1, no. 65 (2002): 214–18.

17. P. C. Molan, "Potential of Honey in the Treatment of Wounds and Burns." *American Journal of Clinical Dermatology* 1, no. 2 (2001): 13–19.

18. Sally Fallon, Pat Connolly, Mary Enig, *Nourishing Traditions* (San Diego: ProMotion Publishing, 1995).

19. Ibid.

20. "Food Data," www.gicare.com.

21. "Food Data," www.calorieking.com.

22. M. R. Ellis and S. Meadows, "What Is the Best Therapy for Constipation in Infants?" *Journal of Family Practice*, August 2002.

23. "Sugar-Free Blues," www.westonaprice.org.

24. P. Guo and D. Clouatre, "Lo Han: A Natural Sweetener Comes of Age," *Whole Foods*, June 2003.

25. M. A. Hossen and Y. Shinmei, "Effect of Lo Han Kuo (Siraitia grosvenori Swingle) on Nasal Rubbing and Scratching Behavior in ICR Mice," *Biological and Pharmaceutical Bulletin* 28, no. 2 (February 2005): 238–41.

26. Fallon, *Nourishing Traditions.*

27. P. Bergner, *The Healing Power of Minerals, Special Nutrients, and Trace Elements* (Prima Lifestyles, 1997).

28. Fallon, *Nourishing Traditions.*

29. E-mail to author dated 06/29/2006 from Adept Solutions, Inc., a Soquel, California company and industry leader in product development and formulation.

30. 21CFR101.4, http://frwebgate2.access.gpo.gov/cgi-bin/waisgate.cgi?WAISdocID =601332263337+1+0+0&WAISaction=retrieve.

31. Fallon, *Nourishing Traditions.*

32. "Agave Syrup," www.aroma-essence.com.

33. Lynn Stephens, "Shake Off the Sugar," www.shakeoffthesugar.net.

34. Burkhard Bilger, "The Search for Sweet: Building a Better Sugar Substitute," *New Yorker*, May 22, 2006.

35. Melanie Warner, "US: Senomyx's Fake Flavors," *New York Times*, April 6, 2005, http://www.corpwatch.org/article.php?id=12053.

36. Pharmaceutical chemist (PhD) and consultant to the food industry who wishes to remain anonymous.

37. K. L. Teff, S. S. Elliott, M. Tschop, T. J. Kieffer, D. Rader, M. Heiman, R. R. Townsend, N. L. Keim, D. D'Alessio, and P. J. Havel, "Dietary Fructose Reduces Circulating Insulin and Leptin, Attenuates Postprandial Suppression of Ghrelin, and Increases Triglycerides in Women," *Journal of Clinical Endocrinology and Metabolism* 6, no. 89 (June 2004): 2963–72.

38. J. P. Bantle, S. Raatz, W. Thomas, and A. Georgopoulo, "Effects of Dietary Fructose on Plasma Lipids in Healthy Subjects," *American Journal of Clinical Nutrition* 5, no. 72 (November 2000): 1128–34.

39. A. M. Puvo, M. A. Mayer, S. Cavallero, A. S. Donoso, and H. A. Peredo, "Fructose Overload Modifies Vascular Morphology and Prostaglandin Production in Rats," *Autonomic and Autacoid Pharmacology* 2, no. 24 (April 2004): 29–35.

40. H. Basciano, L. Federico, and K. Adelli, "Fructose, Insulin Resistance, and Metabolic Dyslipidemia," *Nutrition and Metabolism* 21 1, no. 2 (February 2005): 5.

41. Puvo et al., "Fructose Overload Modifies Vascular Morphology and Prostaglandin Production in Rats."

42. G. L. Kelley, G. Allan, and S. Azhar, "High Dietary Fructose Induces a Hepatic Stress Response Resulting in Cholesterol and Lipid Dysregulation," *Endocrinology* 2, no. 145 (February 2004): 548–55.

43. S. Twetman and C. Stecksen-Blicks, "Effect of Xylitol-Containing Chewing Gums on Lactic Acid Production in Dental Plaque from Caries Active Pre-School Children," *Oral Health and Preventive Dentistry* 3, no. 1 (2003): 195–99.

44. "Sugar Alcohols," www.innvista.com.

45. W. Glinsman, H. Rausquin, and Y. Park, "Evaluation of Health Aspects of Sugars Contained in Carbohydrate Sweeteners," FDA Report of Sugars Task Force, 1986, 39.

46. Ibid.

47. Russ Bianchi, Letter To The Editor Regarding Maltitol. *Nutraceutical World* (March 2002) and interview with Dr. Bianchi.

48. "Naturalose," www.tagatose.com.

49. J. P. Saunders, T. W. Donner, J. H. Sadler, G. V. Levin, and N. G. Makris, "Effects of Acute and Repeated Oral Doses of D-Tagatose on Plasma Uric Acid in Normal and Diabetic Humans," *Regulatory Toxicology and Pharmacology* 29, no. 2, pt. 2 (April 1999): S57–65.

50. Source is a food chemist who wishes to remain anonymous.

ADDITIONAL CHAPTER EIGHT REFERENCES

Rosedale, R., and C. Colman. *The Rosedale Diet*. New York: HarperCollins, 2004.

APPENDIX A

1. A. Sanchez et al., "Role of Sugars in Human Neutrophilic Phagocytosis," *American Journal of Clinical Nutrition* 261 (November 1973): 1180–84; J. Bernstein et al., "Depression of Lymphocyte Transformation Following Oral Glucose Ingestion," *American Journal of Clinical Nutrition* 30 (1997): 613.

2. W. Ringsdorf, E. Cheraskin, and R. Ramsay, "Sucrose, Neutrophilic Phagocytosis and Resistance to Disease," *Dental Survey* 52, no. 12 (1976): 46–48.

3. F. Couzy et al., "Nutritional Implications of the Interaction Minerals," *Progressive Food and Nutrition Science* 17 (1933): 65–87.

4. A. Kozlovsky et al., "Effects of Diets High in Simple Sugars on Urinary Chromium Losses," *Metabolism* 35 (June 1986): 515–18.

5. M. Fields et al., "Effect of Copper Deficiency on Metabolism and Mortality in Rats Fed Sucrose or Starch Diets," *Journal of Clinical Nutrition* 113 (1983): 1335–45.

6. J. Lemann, "Evidence That Glucose Ingestion Inhibits Net Renal Tubular Reabsorption of Calcium and Magnesium," *Journal of Clinical Nutrition* 70 (1976): 236–45.

7. J. Goldman et al., "Behavioral Effects of Sucrose on Preschool Children," *Journal of Abnormal Child Psychology* 14, no. 4 (1986): 565–77.

8. T. W. Jones et al., "Enhanced Adrenomedullary Response and Increased Susceptibility to Neuroglygopenia: Mechanisms Underlying the Adverse Effect of Sugar Ingestion in Children," *Journal of Pediatrics* 126 (February 1995): 171–77.

9. S. Scantoand and J. Yudkin, "The Effect of Dietary Sucrose on Blood Lipids, Serum Insulin, Platelet Adhesiveness and Body Weight in Human Volunteers," *Postgraduate Medicine Journal* 45 (1969): 602–7.

10. M. Albrink and I. H. Ullrich, "Interaction of Dietary Sucrose and Fiber on Serum Lipids in Healthy Young Men Fed High Carbohydrate Diets," *American Journal of Clinical Nutrition* 43 (1986): 419–28; R. Pamplona et al., "Mechanisms of Glycation in Atherogenesis," *Medical Hypotheses* 40, no. 3 (March 1993): 174–81.

11. S. Reiser, "Effects of Dietary Sugars on Metabolic Risk Factors Associated with Heart Disease," *Nutritional Health*, 1985, 203–16.

12. G. F. Lewis and G. Steiner, "Acute Effects of Insulin in the Control of VLDL Production in Humans. Implications for the Insulin-Resistant State," *Diabetes Care* 19, no. 4 (April 1996): 390–93; M. J. Pamplona et al., "Mechanisms of Glycation in Atherogenesis," *Medical Hypotheses* 40 (1990): 174–81.

13. A. Cerami, H. Vlassara, and M. Brownlee, "Glucose and Aging," *Scientific American*, May 1987, 90; A. T. Lee and A. Cerami, "The Role of Glycation in Aging," *Annals of the New York Academy of Science* (663): 63–67.

14. E. Takahashi, *Tohoku University School of Medicine, Wholistic Health Digest*, October 1982, 41:00.

15. Patrick Quillin, "Cancer's Sweet Tooth," *Nutrition Science News*, April 2000; M. Rothkopf, [article title?] *Nutrition* 6, no. 4 (July/Aug. 1990).

16. D. Michaud, "Dietary Sugar, Glycemic Load, and Pancreatic Cancer Risk in a Prospective Study," *Journal of the National Cancer Institute* 94, no. 17 (September 4, 2002): 1293–300.

17. C. J. Moerman et al., "Dietary Sugar Intake in the Etiology of Biliary Tract Cancer," *International Journal of Epidemiology* 2, no. 2 (April 1993): 207–14.

18. The Edell Health Letter, September 1991, 7:1.

19. E. de Stefani, "Dietary Sugar and Lung Cancer: A Case Control Study in Uruguay," *Nutrition and Cancer* 31, no. 2 (1998): 132–37.

20. J. Cornee et al., "A Case-Control Study of Gastric Cancer and Nutritional Factors in Marseille, France," *European Journal of Epidemiology* 11 (1995): 55–65.

21. J. Kelsay et al., "Diets High in Glucose or Sucrose and Young Women," *American Journal of Clinical Nutrition* 27 (1974): 926–36; B. J. Thomas et al., "Relation of Habitual Diet to Fasting Plasma Insulin Concentration and the Insulin Response to Oral Glucose, Human Nutrition," *Clinical Nutrition* 36C, no. 1 (1983): 49–51.

22. William Dufty, *Sugar Blues* (New York: Warner Books, 1975).

23. *Acta Ophthalmologica Scandinavica*, March 2002, 48;25. H. Taub, ed., "Sugar Weakens Eyesight," *VM Newsletter*, May 1986, 06:00.

24. Dufty, *Sugar Blues*.

25. J. Yudkin, *Sweet and Dangerous* (New York: Bantam Books, 1974), 129.

26. Cornee et al., "A Case-Control Study of Gastric Cancer and Nutritional Factors in Marseille, France."

27. P. G. Persson, A. Ahlbom, and G. Hellers, [article title?] *Epidemiology* 3 (1992): 47–52.

28. T. W. Jones et al., "Enhanced Adrenomedullary Response and Increased Susceptibility to Neuroglygopenia."

29. A. T. Lee and A. Cerami, "The Role of Glycation in Aging," *Annals of the New York Academy of Science* 663 (1992): 63–70.

30. E. Abrahamson and A. Peget, *Body, Mind and Sugar* (New York: Avon, 1977).

31. W. Glinsmann, H. Irausquin, and K. Youngmee, "Evaluation of Health Aspects of Sugar Contained in Carbohydrate Sweeteners," FDA Report of Sugars Task Force, 1986, 39; K. K. Makinen et al., "A Descriptive Report of the Effects of a 16-Month Xylitol Chewing Gum Programme Subsequent to a 40-Month Sucrose Gum Programme," *Caries Research* 32, no. 2 (1998): 107–12.

32. Glinsmann et al., "Evaluation of Health Aspects of Sugar Contained in Carbohydrate Sweeteners."

33. N. Appleton, *Healthy Bones* (New York: Avery Penguin Putnam, 1989).

34. H. Keen et al., "Nutrient Intake, Adiposity, and Diabetes," *British Medical Journal* 1:00 (1989): 655–58.

35. L. Darlington, N. W. Ramsey, and J. R. Mansfield, "Placebo Controlled, Blind Study of Dietary Manipulation Therapy in Rheumatoid Arthritis," *Lancet* 8575, no. 1 (February 1986): 236–38.

36. L. Powers, "Sensitivity: You React to What You Eat," *Los Angeles Times*, February 12, 1985; J. Cheng et al., "Preliminary Clinical Study on the Correlation Between Allergic Rhinitis and Food Factors," *Lin Chuang Er Bi Yan Hou Ke Za Zhi* 16, no. 8 (August 2002): 393–96.

37. S. Erlander, "The Cause and Cure of Multiple Sclerosis, The Disease to End Disease," [source?] 1, no. 3 (March 3, 1979): 59–63.

38. W. J. Crook, *The Yeast Connection* (Tennessee: Professional Books, 1984).

39. K. Heaton, "The Sweet Road to Gallstones," *British Medical Journal* 288:00:00 (April 14, 1984): 1103–4; G. Misciagna et al., [article title?] *American Journal of Clinical Nutrition* 69 (1999): 120–26.

40. T. Cleave, *The Saccharine Disease* (New Canaan, CT: Keats Publishing, 1974).

41. Ibid.

42. T. Cleave and G. Campbell, *Diabetes, Coronary Thrombosis and the Saccharine Disease* (Bristol, England: John Wright and Sons, 1960).

43. K. Behall, "Influence of Estrogen Content of Oral Contraceptives and Consumption of Sucrose on Blood Parameters," *Disease Abstracts International* 431437 (1982).

44. L. Tjäderhane and M. A. Larmas, "High Sucrose Diet Decreases the Mechanical Strength of Bones in Growing Rats," *Journal of Nutrition* 128 (1998): 1807–10.

45. [first initial?] Beck, H. Nielsen, O. Pedersen, and S. Schwartz, "Effects of Diet on the Cellular Insulin Binding and the Insulin Sensitivity in Young Healthy Subjects," *Diabetes* 15 (1978): 289–96.

46. "Sucrose Induces Diabetes in Cat," *Federal Protocol* 6, no. 97 (1974).

47. S. Reiser et al., "Effects of Sugars on Indices on Glucose Tolerance in Humans," *American Journal of Clinical Nutrition* 43 (1986): 151–59.

48. *Journal of Clinical Endocrinology and Metabolism*, August 2000.

49. R. Hodges and T. Rebello, "Carbohydrates and Blood Pressure," *Annals of Internal Medicine* 98 (1983): 838–41.

50. D. Behar et al., "Sugar Challenge Testing with Children Considered Behaviorally Sugar Reactive," *Nutritional Behavior* 1 (1984): 277–88.

51. A. Furth and J. Harding, "Why Sugar Is Bad for You," *New Scientist* 44 (September 23, 1989).

52. J. Simmons, "Is the Sand of Time Sugar?" *Longevity* 00:00 (June 1990): 49–53.

53. N. Appleton, *Lick the Sugar Habit* (New York: Avery Penguin Putnam, 1988).

54. Cleave, *The Saccharine Disease*.

55. Ibid.

56. M. J. Pamplona et al., "Mechanisms of Glycation in Atherogenesis," *Medical Hypotheses* 40 (1990): 174–81.

57. O. Vaccaro, K. J. Ruth, and J. Stamler, "Relationship of Postload Plasma Glucose to Mortality with 19 yr Follow up," *Diabetes Care* 10 (October 15, 1992): 328–34; M. Tominaga et al., "Impaired Glucose Tolerance Is a Risk Factor for Cardiovascular Disease, but Not Fasting Glucose," *Diabetes Care* 2, no. 6 (1999): 920–24.

58. A. T. Lee and A. Cerami, *Modifications of Proteins and Nucleic Acids by Reducing Sugars: Possible Role in Aging. Handbook of the Biology of Aging* (New York: Academic Press, 1990).

59. V. M. Monnier, "Nonenzymatic Glycosylation, the Maillard Reaction and the Aging Process." *Journal of Gerontology* 45, no. 4 (1990): 105–10.

60. Cerami et al., "Glucose and Aging."

61. D. G. Dyer et al., "Accumulation of Maillard Reaction Products in Skin Collagen in Diabetes and Aging," *Journal of Clinical Investigation* 93, no. 6 (1993): 421–22.

62. S. Veromann et al., "Dietary Sugar and Salt Represent Real Risk Factors for Cataract Development," *Ophthalmologica* 217, no. 4 (July–August 2003): 302–7.

63. F. S. Goulart, "Are You Sugar Smart?" *American Fitness* 00:00: (March–April 1991): 34–38.

64. Monnier, "Nonenzymatic Glycosylation, the Maillard Reaction and the Aging Process."

65. A. Ceriello, "Oxidative Stress and Glycemic Regulation," *Metabolism* 49, no. 2, suppl. 1 (February 2000): 27–29.

66. Appleton, *Lick the Sugar Habit.*

67. W. Hellenbrand, "Diet and Parkinson's Disease. A Possible Role for the Past Intake of Specific Nutrients. Results from a Self-Administered Food-Frequency Questionnaire in a Case-Control Study," *Neurology* 47, no. 3 (September 1996): 644–50.

68. Goulart, "Are You Sugar Smart?"

69. Ibid.

70. J. Yudkin, S. Kang, and K. Bruckdorfer, "Effects of High Dietary Sugar," *British Journal of Medicine,* November 22, 1980, 1396.

71. N. J. Blacklock, N. J. "Sucrose and Idiopathic Renal Stone," *Nutrition and Health* 5, nos.1–2 (1987): 9-; G. Curhan et al., "Beverage Use and Risk for Kidney Stones in Women," *Annals of Internal Medicine* 28 (1998): 534–40.

72. Goulart, "Are You Sugar Smart?"

73. Ibid.

74. Ibid.

75. Ibid.

76. J. Nash, "Health Contenders," *Essence* 23:00 (January 1992): 79–81.

77. E. Grand, "Food Allergies and Migraine," *Lancet* 1 (1979): 955–59.

78. A. Schauss, *Diet, Crime and Delinquency* (Berkley, CA: Parker House, 1981).

79. R. Molteni et al., "A High-Fat, Refined Sugar Diet Reduces Hippocampal Brain-Derived Neurotrophic Factor, Neuronal Plasticity, and Learning," *NeuroScience* 112, no. 4 (2002): 803–14.

80. L. Christensen, "The Role of Caffeine and Sugar in Depression," *Nutrition Report* 9, no. 3 (March 1991): 17–24.

81. Ibid., 44.

82. J. Yudkin, *Sweet and Dangerous* (New York: Bantam Books, 1974).

83. J. Frey, "Is There Sugar in the Alzheimer's Disease?" *Annales De Biologie Clinique* 59, no. 3 (2001): 253–57.

84. J. Yudkin, "Metabolic Changes Induced by Sugar in Relation to Coronary Heart Disease and Diabetes," *Nutrition and Health* 5, nos.1–2 (1987): 5–8.

85. J. Yudkin and O. Eisa, "Dietary Sucrose and Oestradiol Concentration in Young Men," *Annals of Nutrition and Metabolism* 32, no. 2 (1988): 53–55.
86. *The Edell Health Letter*, September 1991, 7:1.
87. L. Gardner and S. Reiser, "Effects of Dietary Carbohydrate on Fasting Levels of Human Growth Hormone and Cortisol," *Proceedings of the Society for Experimental Biology and Medicine* 169 (1982): 36–40.
88. [author? Article?] *Journal of Advanced Medicine* 7, no. 1 (1994): 51–58.
89. Ceriello, "Oxidative Stress and Glycemic Regulation."
90. [author? Article?] *Postgraduate Medicine* 45 (September 1969): 602–07.
91. C. M. Lenders, "Gestational Age and Infant Size at Birth Are Associated with Dietary Intake Among Pregnant Adolescents," *Journal of Nutrition*, June 1997, 1113–17.
92. Ibid.
93. "Sugar, White Flour Withdrawal Produces Chemical Response," *The Addiction Letter*, July 1992, 04:00; C. Colantuoni et al., "Evidence That Intermittent, Excessive Sugar Intake Causes Endogenous Opioid Dependence," *Obesity Research* 10, no. 6 (June 2002): 478–88; Annual Meeting of the American Psychological Society, Toronto, June 17, 2001, www.mercola.com.
94. Ibid.
95. A. L. Sunehag et al., "Gluconeogenesis in Very Low Birth Weight Infants Receiving Total Parenteral Nutrition," *Diabetes* 48 (1999): 7991–8000.
96. L. Christensen L. et al., "Impact of a Dietary Change on Emotional Distress," *Journal of Abnormal Psychology* 94, no. 4 (1985): 565–79.
97. [name? article?] *Nutrition Health Review*, Fall 1985.
98. D. S. Ludwig et al., "High Glycemic Index Foods, Overeating and Obesity," *Pediatrics* 103, no. 3 (March 1999): 26–32.
99. [author? Article title?] *Pediatrics Research* 38, no. 4 (1995): 539–42; J. L. Berdonces, "Attention Deficit and Infantile Hyperactivity," *Revista de Enfermia* 4, no. 1 (January 2001): 11–14.
100. Blacklock, "Sucrose and Idiopathic Renal Stone."
101. F. Lechin et al., "Effects of an Oral Glucose Load on Plasma Neurotransmitters in Humans," *Neurophychobiology* 26, nos. 1–2 (1992): 4–11.
102. M. Fields, [article title?] *Journal of the American College of Nutrition* 17, no. 4 (August 1998): 317–21.
103. A. I. Arieff, "Veterans Administration Medical Center in San Francisco," *San Jose Mercury*, June 12, 1986.
104. Benjamin P. Sandler, *Diet Prevents Polio* (Milwakuee, WI: The Lee Foundation for Nutritional Research, 1951).
105. Patricia Murphy, "The Role of Sugar in Epileptic Seizures," *Townsend Letter for Doctors and Patients*, May 2001. Murphy is editor of Epilepsy Wellness Newsletter, 1462 West 5th Ave., Eugene, Oregon 97402.
106. N. Stern and M. Tuck, *Pathogenesis of Hypertension in Diabetes Mellitus. Diabetes Mellitus, a Fundamental and Clinical Test*, 2nd ed. (Philadelphia: Lippincott Williams & Wilkins, 2000), 943–57.

107. D. Christansen, "Critical Care: Sugar Limit Saves Lives," *Science News* 159 (June 30, 2001): 404.

108. D. Donnini et al., "Glucose May Induce Cell Death Through a Free Radical-Mediated Mechanism," *Biochemical and Biophysical Research Communications* 219, no. 2 (February 15, YEAR): 412–17.

109. S. Schoenthaler, "The Los Angeles Probation Department Diet-Behavior Program: Am Empirical Analysis of Six Institutional Settings," *Int J Biosocial Res* 5, no. 2 (year?): 88–89.

110. "Gluconeogenesis in Very Low Birth Weight Infants Receiving Total Parenteral Nutrition," *Diabetes* 48, no. 4 (April 1999): 791–800.

111. Glinsmann et al., "Evaluation of Health Aspects of Sugar Contained in Carbohydrate Sweeteners"; Yudkin and Eisa, "Dietary Sucrose and Oestradiol Concentration in Young Men."

Appendix D

1. H. K. Yaggi, A. B. Araujo, and J. B. McKinlay, "Sleep Duration as a Risk Factor for the Development of Type 2 Diabetes," *Diabetes Care* 29, no. 3 (March 2006): 657–61.

Appendix E

1. B. Meehan, *Shell Bed to Shell Midden* (Canberra, Australia: Humanities Press, 1982).

2. K. Hawkes, K. Hill, and J. F. O'Connell, "Why Hunters Gather: Optimal Foraging and the Ache of Eastern Paraguay," *American Ethnologist* 9 (1982): 379–98.

3. The Honey Association, "A Brief History of Honey," www.honeyassociation.com.

4. P. Macinnis, *Bittersweet: The Story of Sugar* (Crows Nest: Allen & Unwin, 2002).

5. Ibid.

6. Ibid.

7. N. Appleton, *Lick the Sugar Habit* (Garden City Park, NY: Avery Publishing Group, 1996).

8. Macinnis, *Bittersweet*.

ABOUT THE AUTHORS

JOSEPH MERCOLA, DO, is a widely renowned and respected physician with over three decades of clinical experience. He is the founder of Mercola.com, the world's most visited natural/alternative health Web site, with over 50,000 pages of health information and over 700,000 subscribers to his free health newsletter.

His Web site's mission is to facilitate the transformation of the fatally flawed conventional medical paradigm to one focused on treating the underlying cause of disease. His mission is to help people understand the true sources of disease, and then to take control of their own health with practical, simple, and inexpensive natural resources.

Dr. Mercola is a *New York Times* best-selling author whose previous books include *Dr. Mercola's Total Health Program* and *The No-Grain Diet.*

He is also the director of the Optimal Wellness Center just outside Chicago, one of the nation's leading natural-health clinics. As an osteopathic physician he first trained in conventional medicine and later received extensive training in natural medicine. He was previously chairman of the department of family practice at St. Alexius Hospital in Schaumburg, Illinois, for five years.

He has been interviewed hundreds of times for his medical, dietary, and health-care industry expertise, including ABC's *World News Tonight,* Fox TV, CNN, *Forbes,* CBS, and NBC.

KENDRA DEGEN PEARSALL, NMD, is a Naturopathic Medical Doctor (a primary care physician specializing in natural medicine) who graduated from Southwest College of Naturopathic Medicine, one of six Council of Naturopathic Medical Education (CNME) accredited, four-year naturopathic medical schools in North America. Dr. Pearsall is the coauthor of *Dr. Mercola's Total Health Cookbook and Program* and the medical editor of *The Hormone Handbook*. She specializes in natural, holistic weight loss, and her weight loss review Web site is Weightloss.WorldEnlightened.com.

If optimizing your health and weight matter to you—and because you are reading this book it is apparent they do—learning your "metabolic type" is one of THE most important steps you need to take.

Everyone is either a "Carb," "Protein," or "Mixed Type," and in the free mini-course you will discover why learning your type is so crucial to your health, and how you can use it to **greatly accelerate your health & weight** improvement right away. You will also discover the fastest and most reliable to learn your type instantly.

In addition, at SweetDeception.com you will instantly receive the new e-report I (Dr. Mercola) recently authored, *The Five "Health Foods" You Should Avoid*, FREE, plus you will be subscribed to the world's #1 most popular and trusted health & wellness newsletter, "Mercola eHealthy News You Can Use," FREE as well!

Learning whether you are a Carb, Protein, or Mixed metabolic type—and how to eat according to that information—is the first key step to:

- **Prevent disease, from "common" illnesses to chronic disease**
- **Avoid premature aging and instead look and feel younger**
- **Reach your ideal weight . . . permanently**
- **Increase your daily energy and ability to stay focused**
- **Live longer and better**

So go to www.sweetdeception.com today and get your metabolic typing email mini-course—and get the bonus report and my health newsletter—all FREE for a limited time!

CPSIA information can be obtained at www.ICGtesting.com
Printed in the USA
LVOW040712170613

338869LV00002B/13/P